101
SWEET AND SAVORY FAT BOMB RECIPES

~~~

By Thomas Daniels
~~~

© **Copyright 2018 by Jamiet- All rights reserved.**

This document is geared towards providing exact and reliable information in regards to the topic and issue covered. The publication is sold with the idea that the publisher is not required to render accounting, officially permitted, or otherwise, qualified services. If advice is necessary, legal or professional, a practiced individual in the profession should be ordered.

- From a Declaration of Principles which was accepted and approved equally by a Committee of the American Bar Association and a Committee of Publishers and Associations.

In no way is it legal to reproduce, duplicate, or transmit any part of this document in either electronic means or in printed format. Recording of this publication is strictly prohibited and any storage of this document is not allowed unless with written permission from the publisher. All rights reserved.

The information provided herein is stated to be truthful and consistent, in that any liability, in terms of inattention or otherwise, by any usage or abuse of any policies, processes, or directions contained within is the solitary and utter responsibility of the recipient reader. Under no circumstances will any legal responsibility or blame be held against the publisher for any reparation, damages, or monetary loss due to the information herein, either directly or indirectly.

Respective authors own all copyrights not held by the publisher.

The information herein is offered for informational purposes solely, and is universal as so. The presentation of the information is without contract or any type of guarantee assurance.

The trademarks that are used are without any consent, and the publication of the trademark is without permission or backing by the trademark owner. All trademarks and brands within this book are for clarifying purposes only and are the owned by the owners themselves, not affiliated with this document.

TABLE OF CONTENTS

CHOCOLATE PEANUT BUTTER FAT BOMBS

Prep Time: 5 minutes
Cooking Time: 30 minutes
Servings: 45 to 50

Nutritional Info (Estimated Amount Per Serving)

- 52 Calories

- 36 Calories from Fat

- 4g Total Fat

- 2.2g Saturated Fat

- 0g Trans Fat

- 0.3g Polyunsaturated Fat

- 0.9g Monounsaturated Fat

- 0mg Cholesterol

- 11mg Sodium

- 20mg Potassium

- 3.4g Total Carbohydrates

- 0.4g Dietary Fiber

- 2.3g Sugars

- 0.9g Protein

INGREDIENTS

- 2-4 tbsp. Agave Nectar or Stevia

- ½ cup almond butter or natural peanut butter (it shouldn't have more than 5 gr of sugar)

- A splash of vanilla extract

- 2-3 tbsp. cocoa powder, unsweetened

- ½ cup virgin coconut oil, organic

DIRECTIONS

1. Over low-heat settings in a large skillet; heat the peanut butter and coconut oil until completely melted. Add the cocoa powder; give everything a good stir.

2. Now, stir in the agave nectar or stevia; stir well until evenly mixed.

3. Remove the skillet immediately from heat & add in the vanilla extract.

4. To make the pouring process easier; transfer the mixture to a spouted cup and then pour approximately ½ tablespoon of the mixture into the silicone candy molds.

5. Refrigerate or freeze until completely set.

6. Remove the set bombs from molds & store them in an air tight container in the fridge. Serve and enjoy.

FUDGE
FAT BOMBS

Prep Time: 35 minutes
Cooking Time: 2 hours
Servings: 30

Nutritional Info (Estimated Amount Per Serving)

- 128 Calories

- 114 Calories from Fat

- 13g Total Fat

- 6.9g Saturated Fat

- 0g Trans Fat

- 1.3g Polyunsaturated Fat

- 3.2g Monounsaturated Fat

- 0mg Cholesterol

- 4.1mg Sodium

- 68mg Potassium

- 2.7g Total Carbohydrates

- 1.3g Dietary Fiber

- 0.5g Sugars

- 2.1g Protein

INGREDIENTS

- ½ cup cocoa powder, unsweetened

- 1 cup almond butter

- ¼ tsp. powdered stevia

- 1/16 tsp. pink Himalayan salt

- 1 cup coconut oil, at room temperature

- 1/3 cup coconut flour

DIRECTIONS

1. Heat the coconut oil in a small pot until completely melted (preferably over medium heat settings) and then and add in the almond butter; mix well.

2. Add the entire dried ingredients together in the same pot; give everything a good stir until combined well.

3. Set aside and let the mixture to slightly cool; taste and feel free to add more of sweetener to taste.

4. Transfer the prepared mixture into a large bowl & then place in a freezer for one and half hours.

5. Once solidified, immediately remove the bowl from freezer. Using clean hands; form approximately 30 balls from the mixture.

6. Place the formed balls on a clean plate or flat tray & place it again into the freezer for a couple of more minutes.

7. Serve and enjoy.

WHITE CHOCOLATE FAT BOMBS

Prep Time: 5 minutes
Cooking Time: 15 minutes
Servings: 8

Nutritional Info (Estimated Amount Per Serving)

- 136 Calories

- 122 Calories from Fat

- 14g Total Fat

- 9.7g Saturated Fat

- 0g Trans Fat

- 0.3g Polyunsaturated Fat

- 2.7g Monounsaturated Fat

- 0mg Cholesterol

- 0.5mg Sodium

- 7.8mg Potassium

- 1.1g Total Carbohydrates

- 0g Dietary Fiber

- 0.7g Sugars

- 0g Protein

INGREDIENTS

- ¼ cup coconut oil (approximately 35 grams)

- 10 drops of vanilla stevia

- ¼ cup cocoa butter (approximately 25 grams)

DIRECTIONS

1. Over low-heat settings or in a double boiler; melt the cocoa butter together with the coconut oil.

2. Once done; remove from the heat & then stir in the stevia drops; stir well.

3. Pour the mixture into the molds and let chill in a refrigerator until hardened, for several minutes.

4. Remove the fat bombs from molds & store them in an air-tight container in a refrigerator until ready to serve.

GLUTEN-FREE BUTTER-CREAM FAT BOMBS

Prep Time: 5 minutes
Cooking Time: 15 minute
Servings: 2

Nutritional Info (Estimated Amount Per Serving)

- 1032 Calories

- 934 Calories from Fat

- 104g Total Fat

- 64g Saturated Fat

- 2.8g Trans Fat

- 4.1g Polyunsaturated Fat

- 27g Monounsaturated Fat

- 272mg Cholesterol

- 827mg Sodium

- 223mg Potassium

- 22g Total Carbohydrates

- 1.1g Dietary Fiber

- 18g Sugars

- 6.9g Protein

INGREDIENTS

For Butter-cream Fat Bombs:

- ¾ cup of each organic grass-fed butter & cream cheese, preferably at room temperature

- 1 tsp. vanilla extract

- 2-6 tbsp. xylitol or Swerve confectioners to taste

For Coating:

- Toasted almonds, chopped roughly

- Dark chocolate

DIRECTIONS

1. Add cream cheese together with vanilla extract & butter to a large-sized bowl. Using an electric mixer; cream the mixture until super smooth and evenly combined. Slowly add in the xylitol or swerve until you get your desired taste. Spoon the mixture into ice tray or molds & freeze until set and hardened.

2. Now, for the chocolate layer: melt chocolate in the microwave or in a water bath. Set aside and let cool at room temperature until easy to handle.

3. Remove the fat bombs from the ice tray or molds and dip each into the melted chocolate using a fork. Transfer the coated fat bombs over a plate lined with parchment. For a thicker coating; repeat these steps; freeze again.

4. Keep frozen or refrigerated until ready to serve.

DELICIOUS PEPPERMINT FAT BOMBS

Prep Time: 10 minutes
Cooking Time: 10 minutes
Servings: 6

Nutritional Info (Estimated Amount Per Serving)

- 194 Calories

- 187 Calories from Fat

- 21g Total Fat

- 17g Saturated Fat

- 0g Trans Fat

- 0.4g Polyunsaturated Fat

- 1.3g Monounsaturated Fat

- 0mg Cholesterol

- 0mg Sodium

- 0.1mg Potassium

- 1.2g Total Carbohydrates

- 0.3g Dietary Fiber

- 0.2g Sugars

- 0.3g Protein

INGREDIENTS

- 1 tbsp. granulated sweetener, any of your choice or to taste

- 125 g melted coconut oil

- 2 tbsp. unsweetened cocoa

- ¼ tsp. peppermint essence

DIRECTIONS

1. Mix the peppermint essence together with melted coconut oil and sweetener.

2. Pour ½ of the mixture into the ice cube trays or silicon cases. Place the trays inside the fridge until a white layer appears on the top.

3. Now, add cocoa powder to the leftover mixture and then pour the mixture over the white layer.

4. Place the trays again in the fridge until completely set.

STRAWBERRY CHEESECAKE FAT BOMBS

Prep Time: 10 minutes
Cooking Time: 2 hours & 20 minutes
Servings: 4

Nutritional Info (Estimated Amount Per Serving)

- 293 Calories

- 257 Calories from Fat

- 29g Total Fat

- 20g Saturated Fat

- 0g Trans Fat

- 0.9g Polyunsaturated Fat

- 4.7g Monounsaturated Fat

- 44mg Cholesterol

- 141mg Sodium

- 96mg Potassium

- 5.1g Total Carbohydrates

- 0.4g Dietary Fiber

- 3.1g Sugars

- 2.8g Protein

INGREDIENTS

- ½ to 1 tbsp. vanilla extract or 1 vanilla bean

- 10 to 15 drops of liquid stevia or 2 tbsp. powdered erythritol

- ¾ cup cream cheese, softened (cut into small pieces)

- ½ cup strawberries, fresh or frozen

- ¼ cup coconut oil or butter, softened

DIRECTIONS

1. Place the coconut oil or butter and cream cheese into a large-sized mixing bowl. Set aside and let rest until softened, for 30 to 60 minutes, at room temperature. Ensure you don't microwave the butter.

2. In the meantime, wash and get rid of the green parts from the fresh or frozen strawberries. Place them in a large bowl; mashing them using a fork.

3. Add the vanilla extract and stevia or powdered erythritol; mix well. Once the strawberries have reached the room temperature; mix them with the cream cheese, softened butter and other leftover ingredients in the bowl.

4. Mix using a food processor or hand whisk until combined well.

5. Spoon the mixture out into candy molds or muffin silicon molds, preferably small-sized. Place the molds in a freezer until set, for approximately 2 hours.

6. After 2 hours, unmold the fat bombs & place them in a container. Let the fat bombs to remain in the freezer until ready to serve.

PEANUT BUTTER CHOCOLATE FAT BOMBS

Prep Time: 15 minute
Cooking Time: 15 minute
Servings: 32

Nutritional Info (Estimated Amount Per Serving)

- 144 Calories

- 118 Calories from Fat

- 13g Total Fat

- 6.5g Saturated Fat

- 0.3g Trans Fat

- 1.2g Polyunsaturated Fat

- 4.1g Monounsaturated Fat

- 19mg Cholesterol

- 96mg Sodium

- 80mg Potassium

- 5.3g Total Carbohydrates

- 1.1g Dietary Fiber

- 2.8g Sugars

- 2.4g Protein

INGREDIENTS

For Peanut Butter Layer

- 4 ounces soft Kerry Gold Butter, salted

- 1 cup peanut butter

- 2 tablespoons Swerve Confectioners or Sukrin Melis Icing Sugar

For Chocolate Layers:

- ½ cup Swerve Confectioners or Sukrin Melis Icing Sugar

- 4 ounces unsweetened baking chocolate

- ½ teaspoon vanilla

- 6 ounces soft Kerry Gold Butter, Salted

- ½ teaspoon Stevia Glycerite

DIRECTIONS

1. Lightly coat the bottom and sides of an 8x8" pan (lined with the parchment paper) with the baking spray.

2. Finely chop the chocolate & melt it in a double boiler.

3. Now, in a medium-sized bowl; put 6 ounces of the butter & sift the powdered sweetener. Using a hand mixer; mix until the sweetener starts to dissolve.

4. Check and then add vanilla together with the stevia glycerite, and melted chocolate to the butter; continue to beat for several minutes, until fluffy & you get mousse like consistency.

5. Spread half of the prepared mixture into the coated pan & then place in the freezer.

6. For the peanut butter layer: Blend the ingredients using a hand

mixer until light and creamy. Spread the entire peanut butter over the chocolate layer & place it into the freezer again until firm slightly, for 5 to 10 minutes.

7. Now, spread the prepared chocolate mixture over the layer of peanut butter & let refrigerate for over-night.

8. The next day, run a sharp knife along the sides of the pan and carefully lift the entire thing by pulling up on the parchment. Using a sharp knife; cut into 32 even-sized pieces & store them in the refrigerator until ready to serve, preferably in an air-tight container.

WHITE CHOCOLATE BUTTER PECAN FAT BOMBS

Prep Time: 15 minutes
Cooking Time: 10 minutes
Servings: 4

Nutritional Info (Estimated Amount Per Serving)

- 677 Calories

- 656 Calories from Fat

- 73g Total Fat

- 37g Saturated Fat

- 0.5g Trans Fat

- 16g Polyunsaturated Fat

- 16g Monounsaturated Fat

- 31mg Cholesterol

- 166mg Sodium

- 137mg Potassium

- 5.6g Total Carbohydrates

- 2g Dietary Fiber

- 0.9g Sugars

- 4.7g Protein

INGREDIENTS

- 2 tbsp. butter

- ¼ tsp. vanilla extract

- 2 tbsp. erythritol, powdered

- A pinch of Stevia

- 2 oz. cocoa butter

- ½ cup pecans or walnuts or hazelnuts, chopped

- 2 tbsp. coconut oil

- A pinch of salt

DIRECTIONS

1. Over moderate heat settings in a small pan; heat coconut oil together with cocoa butter & butter until completely melted, and then turn off the heat settings.

2. Add 2 tbsp. of the powdered erythritol into the melted butter mixture; give everything a good stir until well-combined.

3. Now, add a pinch of salt and then a pinch of Stevia; stir well.

4. Add in the vanilla extract; stir until evenly mixed.

5. Add a couple of chopped pecans into some candy molds or silicone cupcake molds.

6. Evenly pour the white chocolate mix over the nuts into the molds & then immediately place the molds in a freezer.

7. Freeze until set, for half an hour.

8. Serve immediately and enjoy.

CHEESECAKE FAT BOMBS

Prep Time: 15 minutes
Cooking Time: 4 hours & 5 minutes
Servings: 12

Nutritional Info (Estimated Amount Per Serving)

- 221 Calories

- 212 Calories from Fat

- 24g Total Fat

- 17g Saturated Fat

- 0.1g Trans Fat

- 0.6g Polyunsaturated Fat

- 3.5g Monounsaturated Fat

- 28mg Cholesterol

- 89mg Sodium

- 27mg Potassium

- 1.4g Total Carbohydrates

- 0g Dietary Fiber

- 0.8g Sugars

- 1.3g Protein

INGREDIENTS

For Top:

- 2 tsp. erythritol or natvia

- ½ cup coconut oil, refined

- 1 tsp. cocoa powder

For Base:

- 1 tbsp. erythritol or natvia

- 3 ½ tbsp. melted butter

- 1 tsp. vanilla extract

- ¼ cup coconut oil, refined

- 1 cup cream cheese

DIRECTIONS

1. Add cream cheese together with butter in a medium-sized mixing bowl; using an electric mixer; mix until combined well.

2. Once done; add in the vanilla followed by coconut oil and native; mix until well-combined.

3. Now, fill the silicon mini cupcake tray (with 12 sections) approximately ¾ full with the mixture.

4. With the help of a small-sized teaspoon; smooth the top flat and then place in a freezer until fairly hard, for 20 minutes.

5. In the meantime; mix the cocoa powder with the leftover natvia and coconut oil in a large bowl; mix well and then pour this prepared mixture on top of the semi frozen base layer; place it in a freezer again and let freeze for a couple of more hours.

DARK CHOCOLATE CREAM CHEESE FAT BOMBS

Prep Time: 5 minutes
Cooking Time: 20 minutes
Servings: 8

Nutritional Info (Estimated Amount Per Serving)

- 339 Calories

- 249 Calories from Fat

- 28g Total Fat

- 14g Saturated Fat

- 0g Trans Fat

- 2.5g Polyunsaturated Fat

- 8.1g Monounsaturated Fat

- 30mg Cholesterol

- 461mg Sodium

- 250mg Potassium

- 18g Total Carbohydrates

- 2.4g Dietary Fiber

- 12g Sugars

- 6.3g Protein

INGREDIENTS

- ¼ cup plus 2 tbsp. coconut oil

- 8 oz. cream cheese, softened at room temperature

- 1 cup dark chocolate chips

- ½ cup peanut butter

- 1 tsp. kosher salt

DIRECTIONS

1. Line a small-sized baking sheet with the parchment paper in advance. Now, combine the cream cheese together with ¼ cup of coconut oil, peanut butter, and salt in a medium-sized bowl. Beat the mixture using a hand mixer for a couple of minutes, until completely combined. Place the bowl into a freezer and let freeze for 10 to 15 minutes, until slightly firm.

2. When hardened; form golf ball sized balls using a small spoon or a cookie scoop. Place the formed balls in the refrigerator for a couple of more minutes, until harden.

3. In the meantime, prepare the chocolate drizzle: In a microwave safe bowl; thoroughly combine the chocolate chips with the leftover coconut oil & microwave until melted completely, preferably in 30 seconds intervals. Drizzle on top of the peanut butter balls & place them into the refrigerator again for a couple of more minutes, until harden. Serve immediately and enjoy.

NO-BAKE PEANUT BUTTER CHOCOLATE FAT BOMBS

Prep Time: 10 minutes
Cooking Time: 30 minutes
Servings: 4

Nutritional Info (Estimated Amount Per Serving)

- 463 Calories

- 407 Calories from Fat

- 45g Total Fat

- 29g Saturated Fat

- 0.1g Trans Fat

- 5.3g Polyunsaturated Fat

- 6.3g Monounsaturated Fat

- 8.5mg Cholesterol

- 82mg Sodium

- 222mg Potassium

- 25g Total Carbohydrates

- 3.1g Dietary Fiber

- 1.9g Sugars

- 7.5g Protein

INGREDIENTS

- 2 tbsp. heavy cream

- ¼ cup cocoa powder

- 6 tbsp. shelled hemp seeds

- 1 tsp. vanilla extract

- ¼ cup unsweetened coconut, shredded

- 28 drops liquid stevia

- ½ cup coconut oil

- 4 tbsp. peanut butter fit powder

DIRECTIONS

1. Mix the entire dry ingredients together with the coconut oil in a large-sized bowl until you get paste like consistency.

2. Add in the vanilla, liquid stevia, and heavy cream. Mix until slightly creamy and well- combined.

3. Measure the unsweetened shredded coconut out on to a clean plate and then using your hand; roll the balls out & then roll them into the shredded coconut.

4. Place the coated balls over a baking tray and cover them with the parchment paper. Place the tray in a freezer and let freeze for 20 minutes, until completely set.

CHOCOLATE WALNUT FAT BOMBS

Prep Time: 10 minutes
Cooking Time: 25 minutes
Servings: 30

Nutritional Info (Estimated Amount Per Serving)

- 42 Calories

- 32 Calories from Fat

- 3.6g Total Fat

- 2.2g Saturated Fat

- 0g Trans Fat

- 0.6g Polyunsaturated Fat

- 0.5g Monounsaturated Fat

- 0.3mg Cholesterol

- 0.8mg Sodium

- 24mg Potassium

- 3.2g Total Carbohydrates

- 0.4g Dietary Fiber

- 1.6g Sugars

- 0.3g Protein

INGREDIENTS

- 1/3 cup walnut pieces, small-sized, crushed using a food processor (keeping few large pieces to decorate)

- 3.5 ounces dark chocolate, minimum 90% cocoa solids

- 1 tsp. cinnamon

- ¼ cup coconut oil

- 8 drops of stevia

DIRECTIONS

1. Melt coconut oil and chocolate in the microwave.

2. Now, add the walnuts pieces together with stevia, and cinnamon to the melted coconut oil-chocolate mixture.

3. Pour the mixture into the ice cube tray or silicone molds & let freeze until set, for a couple of minutes.

4. Remove the tray or molds from the freezer & place the large pieces of walnut over the top; pressing them slightly.

5. Place the fat bombs again into the fridge and let freeze for 20 more minutes.

NEAPOLITAN FAT BOMBS

Prep Time: 10 minutes
Cooking Time: 30 minutes
Servings: 6

Nutritional Info (Estimated Amount Per Serving)

- 415 Calories
- 395 Calories from Fat
- 44g Total Fat
- 31g Saturated Fat
- 0.8g Trans Fat
- 1.3g Polyunsaturated Fat
- 7.7g Monounsaturated Fat
- 72mg Cholesterol
- 192mg Sodium
- 61mg Potassium
- 13g Total Carbohydrates
- 0.4g Dietary Fiber
- 1.7g Sugars
- 2.2g Protein

INGREDIENTS

- 2 strawberries, medium

- ½ cup sour cream

- 2 tbsp. cocoa powder

- ½ cup cream cheese

- 25 drops of liquid Stevia

- ½ cup butter

- 1 tsp. vanilla extract

- 2 tablespoons erythritol

- ½ cup coconut oil

DIRECTIONS

1. Combine the entire ingredients (except strawberries, vanilla and cocoa powder) together in a bowl, preferably large-sized. Mix well using an immersion blender.

2. Evenly divide the mixture between three separate bowls. Add strawberries to the first bowl, cocoa powder to the second & vanilla to the last one.

3. Now, fill the fat bomb mold with the chocolate mixture; place the molds into a refrigerator and let freeze for half an hour. Repeat with strawberry and vanilla layers.

4. Place the molds again into the refrigerator and let freeze for an hour.

CINNAMON BUTTER FAT BOMBS

Prep Time: 15 minutes
Cooking Time: 40 minutes
Servings: 8

Nutritional Info (Estimated Amount Per Serving)

- 443 Calories

- 414 Calories from Fat

- 46g Total Fat

- 29g Saturated Fat

- 1.9g Trans Fat

- 1.7g Polyunsaturated Fat

- 12g Monounsaturated Fat

- 122mg Cholesterol

- 438mg Sodium

- 25mg Potassium

- 9.7g Total Carbohydrates

- 0.5g Dietary Fiber

- 8.9g Sugars

- 0.6g Protein

INGREDIENTS

- 1 tablespoon cinnamon

- ¼ cup honey or 20 drops of SweetLeaf clear liquid stevia & 1 tbsp. honey

- 1 pound grass-fed butter, preferably salted, at room temperature

- Salt (if using unsalted butter) to taste

- 1 ½ teaspoons vanilla extract

DIRECTIONS

1. Add butter together with vanilla extract, stevia/honey, and cinnamon to the bottom of your food processor. Process on high settings (start with the lowest available settings) for a few minutes until evenly mixed; stopping in-between & scrapping the food processor as required.

2. Now, fill silicone molds with the butter mixture.

3. Freeze for a couple of hours and then carefully remove from molds. Store them in your freezer in an air-tight container. Serve and enjoy.

LOW CARB RED VELVET FAT BOMBS

Prep Time: 10 minutes
Cooking Time: 55 minutes
Servings: 6

Nutritional Info (Estimated Amount Per Serving)

- 360 Calories

- 274 Calories from Fat

- 30g Total Fat

- 19g Saturated Fat

- 0.7g Trans Fat

- 1.2g Polyunsaturated Fat

- 8.1g Monounsaturated Fat

- 73mg Cholesterol

- 180mg Sodium

- 143mg Potassium

- 20g Total Carbohydrates

- 1.2g Dietary Fiber

- 18g Sugars

- 2.6g Protein

INGREDIENTS

- 3.5oz sugar-free dark chocolate (90%)

- 4 drops red food coloring

- 1/3 cup of heavy cream

- 1 tsp. vanilla extract

- 3 tbsp. of Natvia

- 4.4 oz. cream cheese

- 3.5 oz. butter

DIRECTIONS

1. Melt chocolate completely over a pot of boiling water (preferably small-sized) in a heatproof bowl. Ensure you don't let the bowl to touch the simmering water and don't burn the chocolate.

2. In the meantime, mix the leftover ingredients together on medium speed using a Hand Mixer until evenly mixed, for a couple of minutes.

3. With the Mixer still running on the low speed, gradually add chocolate mixture into the leftover ingredients. Mix for a minute or two, on average speed.

4. Add the prepared mix to a Piping Bag & pipe the mix onto a lined tray. Place the tray in a fridge and let chill for 35 to 40 minutes.

5. Now, add heavy cream into a whipping canister & slowly apply it to the prepared fat bombs.

LEMON MACADAMIA FAT BOMBS

Prep Time: 25 minutes
Cooking Time: 25 minutes
Servings: 30

Nutritional Info (Estimated Amount Per Serving)

- 101 Calories

- 92 Calories from Fat

- 10g Total Fat

- 7g Saturated Fat

- 0g Trans Fat

- 0.3g Polyunsaturated Fat

- 2.3g Monounsaturated Fat

- 0mg Cholesterol

- 6.1mg Sodium

- 31mg Potassium

- 2.3g Total Carbohydrates

- 0.7g Dietary Fiber

- 1.4g Sugars

- 0.5g Protein

INGREDIENTS

- 6 ounces coconut oil, organic

- 1 ounce cocoa butter

- A splash of vanilla extract, organic

- 2 ounces coconut cream concentrate, organic

- A pinch of sea salt

- ½ cup shredded coconut unsweetened, organic

- 3 tbsp. organic coconut flour

- Juice & zest of 1 lemon, medium

- 3 tbsp. honeyville blanched almond flour

- ½ cups macadamia nuts

- Liquid Stevia to taste

DIRECTIONS

1. Heat the coconut oil together with cocoa butter and coconut cream concentrate until completely melted, over low heat in a small sauce pan.

2. Now, combine the melted mixture together with the vanilla, flours, stevia, lemon zest/juice, and stevia in a blender. Blend on high settings until combined well, for a minute.

3. Add the macadamia nuts and shredded coconut; pulse a couple of times until lightly chop and combine well.

4. Press the mixture into a silicone mold & place the molds in a refrigerator; let freeze until firm. Serve and enjoy.

CASHEW BUTTER FAT BOMBS

Prep Time: 5 minutes
Cooking Time: 30 minutes
Servings: 12

Nutritional Info (Estimated Amount Per Serving)

- 102 Calories

- 90 Calories from Fat

- 10g Total Fat

- 4.5g Saturated Fat

- 0.2g Trans Fat

- 1.3g Polyunsaturated Fat

- 3.6g Monounsaturated Fat

- 15mg Cholesterol

- 80mg Sodium

- 38mg Potassium

- 2.7g Total Carbohydrates

- 0.2g Dietary Fiber

- 1g Sugars

- 1g Protein

INGREDIENTS

- 6 tbsp. grass-fed butter

- 1 tsp. vanilla extract

- 6 tbsp. cashew butter

- A pinch of sea salt

- ½ tsp. organic honey, raw

DIRECTIONS

1. Line a standard-sized mini muffin tin (with 12 cups) with liners.

2. Now, add grass-fed butter and cashew butter to a microwave safe bowl (preferably medium-sized) & microwave on high settings until the mixture is mostly melted, for a minute.

3. Add the leftover ingredients; give everything a good stir until combined well and no chunks remain.

4. Spoon the prepared mixture evenly into the muffin tin liners.

5. Refrigerate for 40 to 45 minutes or freeze for a minimum period of 10 minutes until semi-soft and chewy. Serve and enjoy.

CHOCOLATE CHERRY FAT BOMBS

Prep Time: 15 minutes
Cooking Time: 1 hours & 15 minutes
Servings: 6

Nutritional Info (Estimated Amount Per Serving)

- 179 Calories

- 146 Calories from Fat

- 16g Total Fat

- 14g Saturated Fat

- 0g Trans Fat

- 0.2g Polyunsaturated Fat

- 0.9g Monounsaturated Fat

- 0mg Cholesterol

- 4.2mg Sodium

- 99mg Potassium

- 9.5g Total Carbohydrates

- 2.8g Dietary Fiber

- 3.2g Sugars

- 1.6g Protein

INGREDIENTS

- ¼ cup melted coconut oil

- ½ tsp. almond extract

- 3 tbsp. cacao powder

- ¾ cup dark sweet cherries, frozen & thawed

- 5 drops of liquid stevia

- ¼ cup melted coconut butter

- ½ tsp. vanilla extract

DIRECTIONS

1. Mix the entire ingredients together (don't mix the dark cherries) in a large bowl until evenly mixed.

2. Now, mash the thawed dark cherries with a fork and mix them (along with their accumulated juices) with the chocolate mixture.

3. Now, fill an ice cube tray with the prepared mixture (approximately 1 tbsp. into each cube) and let freeze until set.

4. Store in an air-tight container in a fridge until ready to serve.

CHOCOLATE ALMOND FAT BOMBS

Prep Time: 5 minutes
Cooking Time: 5 minutes
Servings: 4 persons

Nutritional Info (Estimated Amount Per Serving)

- 804 Calories

- 732 Calories from Fat

- 81g Total Fat

- 53g Saturated Fat

- 0.3g Trans Fat

- 5.6g Polyunsaturated Fat

- 15g Monounsaturated Fat

- 15mg Cholesterol

- 633mg Sodium

- 315mg Potassium

- 18g Total Carbohydrates

- 6.5g Dietary Fiber

- 4g Sugars

- 8.4g Protein

INGREDIENTS

- ½ cup almond butter

- 1 cup skinny coconut oil, melted

- 4 tbsp. cocoa powder, unsweetened

- 1 tablespoon Stevia

- ½ teaspoon vanilla extract

- 2 tbsp. grass-fed butter

- 1 tsp. sea salt or to taste

Optional Ingredients:

- Unsweetened coconut, almonds, berries

DIRECTIONS

1. Mix the entire ingredients together in a food processor; on high settings (starting with the lowest available setting) until smooth, for a minute or two.

2. Pour the prepared mixture into the paper cupcake liners and then sprinkle in the coconut shreds, almonds (sliced or whole), berries, or any of your favorite toppings. If desired, feel free to top each cupcake with a small pinch of sea salt.

3. Place the cupcake lines into a refrigerator and let chill until set. Store in an air-tight container, in the fridge until ready to serve.

PUMPKIN PIE
FAT BOMBS

Prep Time: 5 minutes
Cooking Time: 1 hour & 15 minutes
Servings: 6

Nutritional Info (Estimated Amount Per Serving)

- 168 Calories

- 106 Calories from Fat

- 12g Total Fat

- 10g Saturated Fat

- 0g Trans Fat

- 0.2g Polyunsaturated Fat

- 0.6g Monounsaturated Fat

- 0.9mg Cholesterol

- 20mg Sodium

- 153mg Potassium

- 10g Total Carbohydrates

- 2.8g Dietary Fiber

- 5.6g Sugars

- 7.2g Protein

INGREDIENTS

- 2 tablespoons pumpkin pie spice, organic
- ¼ cup melted coconut butter, organic
- 2 tablespoons gelatin, grass-fed
- 1 scoop Grass Protein Original Flavor
- 2 tablespoon maple syrup, organic
- ½ cup canned pumpkin, organic
- 2 tablespoons melted coconut oil, organic

DIRECTIONS

1. Add the entire ingredients together in a blender. Blend on high settings until smooth, for a minute or two.

2. Pour the mixture into the ice cube molds (preferably silicone) and let freeze for an hour.

3. Now, carefully remove the fat bombs from the molds. Serve & enjoy.

BLACKBERRY LEMON FAT BOMBS

Prep Time: 10 minutes
Cooking Time: 1 hour & 20 minutes
Servings: 8

Nutritional Info (Estimated Amount Per Serving)

- 203 Calories

- 187 Calories from Fat

- 21g Total Fat

- 15g Saturated Fat

- 0g Trans Fat

- 1.4g Polyunsaturated Fat

- 3.1g Monounsaturated Fat

- 0mg Cholesterol

- 26mg Sodium

- 86mg Potassium

- 3.9g Total Carbohydrates

- 0.7g Dietary Fiber

- 1.2g Sugars

- 1.4g Protein

INGREDIENTS

- ½ cup packed blackberries, fresh

- ¼ cup smooth cashew butter

- ½ cup coconut milk

- 1 to 2 tbsp. lemon juice, fresh or to taste

- ½ cup coconut oil, full-fat

DIRECTIONS

1. Over moderate heat settings in a large saucepan; heat the cashew butter together with coconut oil, and coconut milk until just warm & well-combined.

2. Place this mixture either in a blender or food processor; add the lemon juice and blackberries.

3. Taste and feel free to add any of the ingredient more, as required.

4. Evenly pour the prepared mixture into the ice cube tray or mini muffin pan; place the tray in a refrigerator and let chill until hard, for an hour. Serve and enjoy or store them in a refrigerator or freezer, covered until ready to serve.

PEACHES & CREAM FAT BOMBS

Prep Time: 10 minutes
Cooking Time: 30 minutes
Servings: 12

Nutritional Info (Estimated Amount Per Serving)

- 79 Calories

- 72 Calories from Fat

- 8g Total Fat

- 4.8g Saturated Fat

- 0.2g Trans Fat

- 0.3g Polyunsaturated Fat

- 2g Monounsaturated Fat

- 23mg Cholesterol

- 67mg Sodium

- 26mg Potassium

- 1.4g Total Carbohydrates

- 0.1g Dietary Fiber

- 0.8g Sugars

- 0.7g Protein

INGREDIENTS

- 2 ounces peaches, Fresh, finely diced

- 1 ounce softened cream cheese, organic (preferably valley cultured)

- ½ teaspoons peach extract

- 2 tablespoons heavy whipping cream

- ¼ cups powdered Erythritol or swerve confectioners

- 2 tablespoons softened butter

- ¼ teaspoons vanilla extract

- 4 ounces softened Bel Giosio Mascarpone

DIRECTIONS

1. Place a standard-sized silicone cupcake molds (with 12 molds) onto a cookie sheet, small-sized. Ensure that the butter, mascarpone and cream cheese all are soft enough, but not melted. Cut the butter into cubes or slices, place them in a microwave safe bowl and microwave for 10 seconds.

2. Cut the cream cheese into cubes and then add them to the bowl (preferably medium-sized); microwave for a couple of more seconds. Add in the mascarpone & place the bowl into the microwave again for 10 seconds more. Quickly whisk until you get a lump-free & creamy consistency. Add vanilla, peach extract, and sweetener; whisk well and then fold or stir in the diced peaches.

3. Evenly spoon the mixture into the molds; smoothing the tops with back of a large spoon. Place the tray into a freezer; let freeze for a couple of hours.

4. Once they are firm, carefully remove the fat-bombs from the molds & place them in an air-tight container or in a large re-sealable bag in a refrigerator. Serve and enjoy.

GLUTEN-FREE NUTTY COCONUT FAT BOMBS

Prep Time: 15 minutes
Cooking Time: 20 minutes
Servings: 15

Nutritional Info (Estimated Amount Per Serving)

- 159 Calories
- 115 Calories from Fat
- 13g Total Fat
- 3g Saturated Fat
- 0g Trans Fat
- 3.3g Polyunsaturated Fat
- 5.8g Monounsaturated Fat
- 0.5mg Cholesterol
- 119mg Sodium
- 181mg Potassium
- 8.6g Total Carbohydrates
- 3.4g Dietary Fiber
- 3.7g Sugars
- 4.7g Protein

INGREDIENTS

- 2 tbsp. chia seeds

- 1 ½ cups walnuts or any nut of your choice

- 2 tbsp. almond butter or any nut butter of your choice

- ½ cup coconut, shredded

- 2 tbsp. hemp seeds

- ¼ cup plus 1 tbsp. coconut butter

- 1 tbsp. maple syrup

- 2 tbsp. flax meal

- ½ tsp. vanilla bean powder

- 1 teaspoon cinnamon

- 2 tbsp. cacao nibs

- ¼ tsp. kosher salt

For The Chocolate Drizzle:

- ½ tsp. coconut oil

- 1 oz. chocolate, unsweetened or bittersweet, chopped

DIRECTIONS

1. Combine the entire ingredients (don't add the cacao nibs) together in the bowl of your food processor. Pulse on high settings (starting with the lowest available setting) until the mixture begins to break down, for a couple of minutes. Don't worry; if it becomes powdery & stick together; it would still be crumbly.

2. Continue to process until the mixture easily sticks together and oils begin to release a bit; don't over process. Feel free to add a tablespoon more of maple syrup or coconut butter, if the mixture seems to be dry. Once the mixture starts sticking together, add in the cacao nibs; pulse until just incorporated.

3. Divide the mixture evenly into pieces using a small tablespoon scoop or a cookie scoop. Form balls from the pieces using your hands; placing the on a clean plate.

4. Now, for chocolate drizzle: Melt the chocolate together with coconut oil for half a minute to a minute in the microwave, if desired. Drizzle the mixture on top of the prepared balls & place in the freezer or fridge until firm up.

5. Serve and enjoy or store them in the freezer or refrigerator, preferably in an airtight container.

COCONUT ALMOND FAT BOMBS

Prep Time: 5 minutes
Cooking Time: 25 minutes
Servings: 15

Nutritional Info (Estimated Amount Per Serving)

- 106 Calories

- 70 Calories from Fat

- 7.8g Total Fat

- 5.7g Saturated Fat

- 0g Trans Fat

- 0.2g Polyunsaturated Fat

- 1.6g Monounsaturated Fat

- 15mg Cholesterol

- 49mg Sodium

- 76mg Potassium

- 6.3g Total Carbohydrates

- 1.2g Dietary Fiber

- 2.9g Sugars

- 3.5g Protein

INGREDIENTS

- 1.7 ounces butter, unsalted

- ¾ tsp. cardamom

- 14 ounces ricotta

- ½ tsp. vanilla extract, unsweetened

- 1 tbsp. psyllium husk

- 1/3 cup coconut, shredded

- 1 scoop of stevia

For Rolling:

- Almonds

- Coconut oil

- Spare coconut, shredded

DIRECTIONS

1. Heat the unsalted butter over low-heat settings in a large pan.

2. Once melted; add in the ricotta; giving everything a good stir until ricotta completely melts.

3. Slowly add 1/3 cup of shredded coconut and a tiny scoop of stevia; mix well.

4. Add psyllium husk; give everything a good stir until evenly mixed.

5. Now, add in the vanilla extract and cardamom; continue to mix until the ingredients begin to form a dough ball, for a couple of minutes.

6. Turn the heat off & set the mixture aside. Let cool at room temperature for 10 minutes.

7. In the meantime; set up a plate or tray. A plate or tray with baking paper over the top.

8. Once you can handle the mixture easily; coat your fingertips lightly with the coconut oil & roll a small quantity into a ball; pressing an almond inside the ball or roll into the shredded coconut & place the coated ball on the plate. Place in a refrigerator or fridge and let chill until set. Serve and enjoy.

PEANUT BUTTER CHOCOLATE CHIP CHEESECAKE FAT BOMBS

Prep Time: 10 minutes
Cooking Time: 55 minutes
Servings: 12

Nutritional Info (Estimated Amount Per Serving)

- 441 Calories

- 334 Calories from Fat

- 37g Total Fat

- 9.4g Saturated Fat

- 0.1g Trans Fat

- 7.5g Polyunsaturated Fat

- 15g Monounsaturated Fat

- 13mg Cholesterol

- 343mg Sodium

- 410mg Potassium

- 18g Total Carbohydrates

- 3.9g Dietary Fiber

- 6.4g Sugars

- 15g Protein

INGREDIENTS

- 1-2 tbsp. xylitol

- 1 package of cream cheese

- 6-8 tbsp. peanut butter

- 1 tbsp. vanilla

- 2 tbsp. butter, grass-fed

- 1 package of dark chocolate chips (9 oz.)

DIRECTIONS

1. Combine the entire ingredients (don't add the chocolate chips) together in a large bowl until evenly mixed, using a hand mixer.

2. Now, stir in the chocolate chips.

3. Form round balls from the mixture or put the prepared dough into a silicone candy mold; place in a freezer for a couple of hours.

4. Serve and enjoy.

MOCHA FAT BOMBS

Prep Time: 15 minutes
Cooking Time: 15 minutes
Servings: 24

Nutritional Info (Estimated Amount Per Serving)

- 64 Calories

- 61 Calories from Fat

- 6.8g Total Fat

- 4.8g Saturated Fat

- 0g Trans Fat

- 0.1g Polyunsaturated Fat

- 0.6g Monounsaturated Fat

- 13mg Cholesterol

- 50mg Sodium

- 11mg Potassium

- 0.5g Total Carbohydrates

- 0g Dietary Fiber

- 0.4g Sugars

- 0.3g Protein

INGREDIENTS

- 2 espresso shots

- 3 oz. cream cheese, softened

- 2 tbsp. heavy whipping cream

- 1 scoop of MCT Oil Powder

- 2 tbsp. monk fruit sweetener

- 5 tbsp. softened Kerrygold butter, unsalted

- 4 tbsp. coconut oil

- ½ scoop of Chocolate Sea Salt

DIRECTIONS

1. Melt butter together with coconut oil, espresso, cream cheese & heavy whipping cream in a double boiler.

2. Remove the bowl from heat & add in the leftover ingredients. Mix the ingredients together until combined well, using a hand mixer.

3. Scoop the mixture out into the silicone mold.

4. Freeze for a couple of hours until set.

5. Once done, carefully remove the fat bombs from the silicone mold. Serve and enjoy.

DELICIOUS DARK CHOCOLATE FAT BOMBS

Prep Time: 15 minutes
Cooking Time: 30 minutes
Servings: 12

Nutritional Info (Estimated Amount Per Serving)

- 173 Calories

- 143 Calories from Fat

- 16g Total Fat

- 13g Saturated Fat

- 0g Trans Fat

- 0.3g Polyunsaturated Fat

- 1.1g Monounsaturated Fat

- 0.2mg Cholesterol

- 25mg Sodium

- 36mg Potassium

- 6.1g Total Carbohydrates

- 1.1g Dietary Fiber

- 3.9g Sugars

- 1.7g Protein

INGREDIENTS

- ¾ cup coconut oil, melted and divided

- 1 tbsp. vanilla Torani syrup, sugar-free

- ¼ cup dark cocoa powder

- Unsweetened coconut flakes, chopped nuts, optional

- ¼ cup peanut butter powder

DIRECTIONS

1. Line a standard-sized mini muffin pan (with 12 cups) with papers.

2. Now, melt the coconut oil in the microwave until the oil is liquid, for a minute (preferably in a 2 cup liquid measuring cup).

3. Add ¼ cup of the melted coconut oil into 2 small-sized mixing bowls; reserving ¼ cup.

4. Add the cocoa powder to a small-sized bowl; continue to mix until completely smooth. This is the time to add the sugar free Torani syrup as well. Distribute the cocoa mixture evenly among the mini muffin pan; adding 1 tbsp. of the mixture to each fat bomb. Now, place the muffin pan into the refrigerator and let chill until harden.

5. Combine peanut butter powder with ¼ cup of the reserved melted coconut oil in a small bowl until smooth. Evenly divide mixture over the chocolate in muffin pan. Refrigerate the pan again until hard.

6. Evenly divide the reserved melted coconut oil on top of the peanut butter layer or add coconut flakes/chopped nuts and let refrigerate until hardened.

7. Carefully remove the bombs from muffin pan; store them in an air-tight baggies or container in the refrigerator until ready to serve.

ALMOND PISTACHIO FAT BOMBS

Prep Time: 5 minutes
Cooking Time: 30 minutes
Servings: 36

Nutritional Info (Estimated Amount Per Serving)

- 150 Calories

- 144 Calories from Fat

- 16g Total Fat

- 12g Saturated Fat

- 0g Trans Fat

- 0.4g Polyunsaturated Fat

- 2.2g Monounsaturated Fat

- 3.6mg Cholesterol

- 14mg Sodium

- 50mg Potassium

- 1.9g Total Carbohydrates

- 1.2g Dietary Fiber

- 0.6g Sugars

- 0.7g Protein

INGREDIENTS

- ¼ tsp. pure almond extract

- 1 cup roasted almond butter, all natural

- ½ cup cacao butter, chopped finely & melted

- 1 cup creamy coconut butter

- ½ cup coconut milk, full-fat, chilled for overnight

- 1 cup firm coconut oil

- ¼ cup ghee

- 2 tsp. chai spice

- ¼ cup shelled pistachios, raw, chopped

- 1 tbsp. vanilla extract, pure

- ¼ tsp. Himalayan salt

DIRECTIONS

1. Lightly grease & line a square baking pan (9") with the parchment paper. For easy unmolding; leaving a little bit hanging on both the sides. Set aside. Now, over low heat settings in a small saucepan; melt the cacao butter, stirring often; set aside.

2. Add the entire ingredients (don't add shelled pistachios and cacao butter) together into a large mixing bowl; mix well using a hand mixer until the mixture turns light & airy and the ingredients are combined well.

3. Now, pour the kept-aside melted cacao butter into the almond mixture; continue to mix until incorporated well, on low speed. Transfer the mixture to prepared pan; evenly spread & then sprinkle chopped pistachios over the top.

4. Refrigerate for 4 hours or for overnight, until completely set.

MOCK PAYDAY
FAT BOMBS

Prep Time: 10 minutes
Cooking Time: 10 minutes
Servings: 16

Nutritional Info (Estimated Amount Per Serving)

- 49 Calories

- 44 Calories from Fat

- 4.9g Total Fat

- 3.7g Saturated Fat

- 0.1g Trans Fat

- 0.1g Polyunsaturated Fat

- 0.6g Monounsaturated Fat

- 4mg Cholesterol

- 24mg Sodium

- 12mg Potassium

- 0.7g Total Carbohydrates

- 0.1g Dietary Fiber

- 0.1g Sugars

- 1.1g Protein

INGREDIENTS

- 2 tbsp. melted butter, salted

- 1 tbsp. whey protein powder

- A dash each of maple extracts and vanilla

- 2 doonks pure stevia extract powder

- A small dash of salt, if required

- 2 tbsp. defatted peanut flour

- Peanuts

- ¼ cup refined coconut oil, melted

DIRECTIONS

1. Stir the entire ingredients (don't add peanuts and salt) together in a large bowl. Taste & add a small pinch of salt, if required.

2. Transfer the prepared candy mixture into the molds. Sprinkle peanuts over the top. Freeze for half an hour to an hour, until hard. Carefully remove the fat-bombs from molds.

3. Store in an air-tight container, in a freezer until ready to serve.

ALMOND BUTTER
FAT BOMBS

Prep Time: 5 minutes
Cooking Time: 5 minutes
Servings: 6

Nutritional Info (Estimated Amount Per Serving)

- 158 Calories

- 135 Calories from Fat

- 15g Total Fat

- 7.9g Saturated Fat

- 0g Trans Fat

- 1.6g Polyunsaturated Fat

- 4g Monounsaturated Fat

- 0mg Cholesterol

- 6.2mg Sodium

- 78mg Potassium

- 4.2g Total Carbohydrates

- 1.5g Dietary Fiber

- 0.5g Sugars

- 2.7g Protein

INGREDIENTS

- ¼ cup Erythritol or powdered swerve

- 2 tbsp. cacao powder

- ¼ cup unrefined coconut oil

- ¼ cup almond butter

DIRECTIONS

1. Mix coconut oil together with almond butter in a medium-sized bowl

2. Microwave for a couple of seconds. Give everything a good stir until completely smooth

3. Now, add in the cacao powder and erythritol; stir well

4. Transfer the prepared mixture into the silicone molds & refrigerate for half an hour to an hour, until firm.

CINNAMON BUN
FAT BOMB BARS

Prep Time: 5 minutes
Cooking Time: 20 minutes
Servings: 2

Nutritional Info (Estimated Amount Per Serving)

- 366 Calories

- 268 Calories from Fat

- 30g Total Fat

- 23g Saturated Fat

- 0g Trans Fat

- 1.4g Polyunsaturated Fat

- 4g Monounsaturated Fat

- 0mg Cholesterol

- 122mg Sodium

- 217mg Potassium

- 24g Total Carbohydrates

- 5.5g Dietary Fiber

- 16g Sugars

- 3g Protein

INGREDIENTS

- 1/8 tsp. cinnamon

- ½ cup creamed coconut, cut into small chunks

For First Icing:

- 1 tbsp. almond butter

- 1 tbsp. extra virgin coconut oil (don't melt the oil)

For Second Icing:

- ½ tsp. cinnamon

- 1 tbsp. almond butter or extra virgin coconut oil

DIRECTIONS

1. Line a mini loaf pan or a dish with the muffin liners.

2. Now, mix coconut cream together with cinnamon using your hands in a medium-sized bowl. Pat the mixture into the loaf pan (filling 2 sections) or dish.

3. For First Icing: Whisk the almond butter together with coconut oil in a separate bowl using a whisk. Spread this mixture on top of the creamed coconut and then place the bars in a freezer for a couple of minutes.

4. For Second Icing: Mix the icing together in a large bowl using a whisk. Drizzle over the bars; freeze again.

5. Cut the prepared bars into small chunks using a sharp knife.

TEMPTING CHOCOLATE WALNUT FAT BOMBS

Prep Time: 10 minutes
Cooking Time: 10 minutes
Servings: 14

Nutritional Info (Estimated Amount Per Serving)

- 112 Calories
- 102 Calories from Fat
- 11g Total Fat
- 7.6g Saturated Fat
- 0g Trans Fat
- 1.5g Polyunsaturated Fat
- 1.2g Monounsaturated Fat
- 0mg Cholesterol
- 0.8mg Sodium
- 18mg Potassium
- 1.9g Total Carbohydrates
- 0.6g Dietary Fiber
- 0.1g Sugars
- 1g Protein

INGREDIENTS

- 1 tbsp. granulated sweetener or to taste

- 25 g unsweetened cocoa powder

- 2 tbsp. tahini paste

- 125 g coconut oil

For Garnish:

- 25 g walnut halves

DIRECTIONS

1. Over low-heat settings in a large pan; heat the coconut oil until completely melted.

2. Now, add the remaining ingredients (don't add the walnuts); set aside and let cool slightly.

3. Pour the mixture into the ice cube trays & refrigerate for half an hour to an hour, until set but not completely set.

4. Once done, place half of the walnut over each fat bomb.

SEA SALTED CHOCOLATE FAT BOMB

Prep Time: 15 minutes
Cooking Time: 10 minutes
Servings: 8

Nutritional Info (Estimated Amount Per Serving)

- 353 Calories

- 343 Calories from Fat

- 38g Total Fat

- 27g Saturated Fat

- 0.8g Trans Fat

- 1.2g Polyunsaturated Fat

- 7.2g Monounsaturated Fat

- 68mg Cholesterol

- 741mg Sodium

- 34mg Potassium

- 2g Total Carbohydrates

- 0.4g Dietary Fiber

- 0.9g Sugars

- 1.4g Protein

INGREDIENTS

- 1/3 cup cream cheese

- 1 tsp. cinnamon

- ½ cup sunflower butter

- 3 tbsp. butter, grass-fed

- ½ cup heavy whipping cream

- 2 tbsp. cocoa powder

- 1 tsp. vanilla

- 2 tsp. coarse sea salt

- ½ cup coconut oil

DIRECTIONS

1. Whip the heavy whipping cream for a couple of minutes, until soft peaks form and then fold in the vanilla.

2. Place coconut oil together with sun-butter, butter, cocoa powder, cinnamon, and Cream Cheese into the food processor; process on high settings (starting with the lowest available speed) until smooth

3. Gently fold the sun-butter mixture into the whipped cream until combined well.

4. Pipe the mixture into silicone molds & then sprinkle coarse sea salt over the top. Transfer the molds into a freezer and let freeze for several hours or for overnight.

TASTY GINGER
FAT BOMBS

Prep Time: 5 minutes
Cooking Time: 5 minutes
Servings: 10

Nutritional Info (Estimated Amount Per Serving)

- 133 Calories

- 125 Calories from Fat

- 14g Total Fat

- 12g Saturated Fat

- 0g Trans Fat

- 0.2g Polyunsaturated Fat

- 0.8g Monounsaturated Fat

- 0mg Cholesterol

- 3.7mg Sodium

- 55mg Potassium

- 2.4g Total Carbohydrates

- 1.6g Dietary Fiber

- 0.8g Sugars

- 0.7g Protein

INGREDIENTS

- 25 g coconut unsweetened, shredded or desiccated

- 1 tsp. granulated sweetener or to taste

- 75 g of each coconut oil & coconut butter, softened

- 1 tsp. ginger powder

DIRECTIONS

1. Mix the entire ingredients together in a large-sized pouring jug for a couple of minutes, until the granulated sweetener is completely dissolved.

2. Now, transfer the mixture into silicon molds and refrigerate for a couple of minutes.

LOW-CARB CHOCOLATE COCONUT FAT BOMBS

Prep Time: 15 minutes
Cooking Time: 15 minutes
Servings: 20

Nutritional Info (Estimated Amount Per Serving)

- 137 Calories
- 122 Calories from Fat
- 14g Total Fat
- 11g Saturated Fat
- 0g Trans Fat
- 0.2g Polyunsaturated Fat
- 1.4g Monounsaturated Fat
- 0.3mg Cholesterol
- 4.3mg Sodium
- 52mg Potassium
- 3.9g Total Carbohydrates
- 1.6g Dietary Fiber
- 1.8g Sugars
- 0.9g Protein

INGREDIENTS

For Coconut Candies:

- ½ cup shredded coconut, unsweetened
- 3 tbsp. Swerve Sweetener, powdered
- ½ cup Kelapo coconut oil
- ½ cup coconut butter

FOR CHOCOLATE TOPPING:

- ¼ cup Swerve Sweetener, powdered
- 1 ½ ounces cocoa butter
- ¼ cup cocoa powder
- 1 ounce chocolate, unsweetened
- ¼ tsp. vanilla extract

DIRECTIONS

For Candies:

1. Line a standard-sized mini-muffin pan with approximately 20 mini paper liners.

2. Now, over low-heat settings in a small-sized saucepan; combine the coconut oil together with coconut butter. Give everything a good stir until smooth and melted, then stir in sweetener and shredded coconut until combined well.

3. Evenly divide the prepared mixture among mini muffin cups & freeze for half an hour, until firm.

For Chocolate Coating:

1. Combine unsweetened chocolate with cocoa butter over a pan of simmering water in a large bowl (ensure that the bowl don't touch the water). Give everything a good stir until completely melted.

2. Now, stir in the sifted powdered sweetener and then add the cocoa powder; stir well until completely smooth.

3. Remove the bowl immediately from heat & then stir in the vanilla extract.

4. The next step would be to spoon the chocolate topping on top of the chilled coconut candies. Let set for several minutes.

5. Serve and enjoy.

EASY VANILLA FAT BOMBS

Prep Time: 15 minutes
Cooking Time: 50 minutes
Servings: 14

Nutritional Info (Estimated Amount Per Serving)

- 139 Calories

- 135 Calories from Fat

- 15g Total Fat

- 7.6g Saturated Fat

- 0g Trans Fat

- 0.3g Polyunsaturated Fat

- 6.1g Monounsaturated Fat

- 0mg Cholesterol

- 1.7mg Sodium

- 35mg Potassium

- 5.3g Total Carbohydrates

- 0.8g Dietary Fiber

- 0.5g Sugars

- 0.8g Protein

INGREDIENTS

- 1 cup unsalted macadamia nuts

- 2 tbsp. Swerve or powdered Erythritol

- ¼ cup grass-fed butter or coconut oil

- 10 to 15 drops of Stevia extract

- 2 tsp. vanilla extract, sugar-free or 1 vanilla bean

- ¼ cup extra virgin coconut oil

DIRECTIONS

1. Pulse the macadamia nuts in a blender until smooth (starting with the lowest available setting).

2. Mix with melted coconut oil and softened butter.

3. Add in the vanilla extract, stevia and powdered Erythritol; mix well until evenly combined.

4. Pour the prepared mixture into an ice cube tray or mini muffin forms. Place the tray inside the fridge and let chill for half an hour, until set.

5. When done; serve and enjoy.

DARK CHOCOLATE RASPBERRY FAT BOMBS

Prep Time: 25 minutes
Cooking Time: 1 hour & 35 minutes
Servings: 14

Nutritional Info (Estimated Amount Per Serving)

- 177 Calories

- 135 Calories from Fat

- 15g Total Fat

- 8.7g Saturated Fat

- 0g Trans Fat

- 0.8g Polyunsaturated Fat

- 4.4g Monounsaturated Fat

- 0.7mg Cholesterol

- 19mg Sodium

- 87mg Potassium

- 16g Total Carbohydrates

- 2.3g Dietary Fiber

- 4.8g Sugars

- 1.7g Protein

INGREDIENTS

For Homemade Chocolate:

- 3 tbsp. coconut oil, extra virgin

- ½ cup cocoa butter

- 4.2 oz. unsweetened dark chocolate, 100% cacao

- ½ - ¾ cup powdered Swerve or Erythritol or to taste

- 1 tsp. unsweetened vanilla extract or 1 vanilla bean; cut length-wise & scrapping the seeds out

- ⅓ cup Dutch process cocoa powder or raw cacao powder

- 20 to 25 drops of Stevia extract or to taste, optional

For Topping:

- 28 almonds

- 1 ½ cup raspberries, fresh or frozen

DIRECTIONS

1. Roast the almonds over moderate heat settings in a large pan for 5 to 7 minutes.

2. Place a piece of roasted almond into each raspberry; spreading over a clean tray & place in the freezer; let chill for an hour.

3. Measure the unsweetened chocolate, cocoa butter & coconut oil. Fill a pot with water & place a bowl over it; bring everything together to a boil (preferably over low heat settings and ensure the bowl doesn't touch the water.

4. Place the unsweetened chocolate, cocoa butter and coconut oil into the bowl & let melt; continue to stir every now and then.

5. In the meantime, powder the Swerve or Erythritol in a blender.

6. Once the chocolate mixture melts, add in the unsweetened cacao, powdered Erythritol, vanilla seeds and stevia; continue to mix the ingredients until combined well & set aside

7. Place a small-sized muffin paper cups on a baking tray & pour approximately 1 tbsp. of the chocolate into each of them

8. Add two frozen raspberries that are filled with the almonds into every cup.

9. Pour a tablespoon of more chocolate on top of them; ensure that you completely cover the raspberries.

10. Place in the fridge and let chill until set, for half an hour.

11. Store the fat bombs in an air-tight container in the fridge for up to 3 days. Serve and enjoy.

BLUEBERRY FAT BOMBS

Prep Time: 5 minutes
Cooking Time: 1 hour & 25 minutes
Servings: 24

Nutritional Info (Estimated Amount Per Serving)

- 125 Calories

- 115 Calories from Fat

- 13g Total Fat

- 9.5g Saturated Fat

- 0.2g Trans Fat

- 0.3g Polyunsaturated Fat

- 1.9g Monounsaturated Fat

- 15mg Cholesterol

- 46mg Sodium

- 15mg Potassium

- 2.7g Total Carbohydrates

- 0.1g Dietary Fiber

- 2.4g Sugars

- 0.4g Protein

INGREDIENTS

- 9/10 cup blueberries (approximately 1 scant)

- ¾ cup coconut oil

- 4 oz butter (approximately 1 stick)

- ¼ cup coconut cream

- 4 oz. cream cheese, softened

- Preferred Sweetener to taste

DIRECTIONS

1. Place coconut cream together with softened cream cheese & berries in a blender or food processor; puree on high settings until smooth, for a minute or two.

2. Now, over low heat settings in a large saucepan; heat the coconut oil and butter & completely melted. Let slightly cool for a couple of minutes & then add them to the blender/food processor as well. Puree on high settings again until smooth.

3. Slowly add the sweetener; give everything a good stir. Taste & adjust the amount of sweetener to your preference. Transfer the mixture to a pitcher or spouted measuring cup & pour the mixture gently into the molds.

4. Place in the freezer & let freeze for an hour, until set.

5. Once done; carefully remove the fat-bombs from the molds. Serve and enjoy.

ICE-CREAM AKA FROZEN FAT BOMB

Prep Time: 20 minutes
Cooking Time: 55 minutes
Servings: 8

Nutritional Info (Estimated Amount Per Serving)

- 373 Calories

- 347 Calories from Fat

- 39g Total Fat

- 26g Saturated Fat

- 0.8g Trans Fat

- 1.6g Polyunsaturated Fat

- 7.8g Monounsaturated Fat

- 180mg Cholesterol

- 117mg Sodium

- 55mg Potassium

- 15g Total Carbohydrates

- 0g Dietary Fiber

- 1.4g Sugars

- 3.1g Protein

INGREDIENTS

- 25-30 drops of Stevia extract (Vanilla/Clear)

- 4 egg yolks, large, organic or free-range

- 2 tbsp. vanilla extract, home-made or 2 vanilla beans

- ¼ cup powdered Erythritol

- 1 cup heavy whipping cream or coconut milk, at room temperature

- ½ cup butter, grass-fed, at room temperature

- 2 eggs, large, organic or free-range; yolks separated from the whites

- ½ cup extra virgin coconut oil, at room temperature

DIRECTIONS

1. Mix the coconut oil together with vanilla extract, butter, stevia and powdered Erythritol in a large bowl.

2. Slowly add in the whole eggs and egg yolks; blending and processing after each addition until completely smooth.

3. Add the coconut milk; continue to blend.

4. Scoop the mixture out into the ice-cream maker & process as per the directions provided by the manufacturer

5. Remove from the ice-cream maker when you reach the half way mark and pulse using an immersion blender until completely smooth.

6. Place it again to the ice-cream maker; continue the process until done. Feel free to pulse with the immersion blender one more time; if lumps remain. Serve immediately and enjoy.

CREAMSICLE FAT BOMBS

Prep Time: 5 minutes
Cooking Time: 3 hours & 15 minutes
Servings: 10

Nutritional Info (Estimated Amount Per Serving)

- 177 Calories
- 171 Calories from Fat
- 19g Total Fat
- 14g Saturated Fat
- 0.2g Trans Fat
- 0.5g Polyunsaturated Fat
- 2.8g Monounsaturated Fat
- 25mg Cholesterol
- 39mg Sodium
- 26mg Potassium
- 3.2g Total Carbohydrates
- 0g Dietary Fiber
- 0.8g Sugars
- 1g Protein

INGREDIENTS

- 4 oz. cream cheese
- ½ cup coconut oil
- 1 tsp. orange vanilla Mio
- ½ cup heavy whipping cream
- 10 drops of liquid stevia

DIRECTIONS

1. Blend the entire ingredients together using an immersion blender in a large bowl. Microwave until soften, if required.

2. Now, spread the prepared mixture evenly into a silicone tray; place the tray in a freezer and let freeze for a couple of hours, until set.

3. Carefully remove the fat-bombs from the tray & store in an air-tight container in a freezer until ready to serve.

MAPLE PECAN FAT BOMBS

Prep Time: 5 minutes
Cooking Time: 25 minutes
Servings: 12

Nutritional Info (Estimated Amount Per Serving)

- 319 Calories

- 272 Calories from Fat

- 30g Total Fat

- 11g Saturated Fat

- 0g Trans Fat

- 6.3g Polyunsaturated Fat

- 11g Monounsaturated Fat

- 0mg Cholesterol

- 3.9mg Sodium

- 208mg Potassium

- 16g Total Carbohydrates

- 4.6g Dietary Fiber

- 5.5g Sugars

- 4.6g Protein

INGREDIENTS

- ¼ cup maple syrup

- 2 cups pecan halves

- ½ cup golden flaxseed meal

- 1 cup almond flour

- ½ cup coconut oil

- 25 drops of liquid stevia

- ½ cup shredded coconut, unsweetened

DIRECTIONS

1. Preheat your oven at 350 F in advance and then toast pecans in the preheated oven for 6 to 8 minutes. Remove & crush them using a rolling pin in a large, re-sealable plastic bag.

2. Add the entire dry ingredients together to a large bowl; mix well.

3. Now, add the wet ingredients; mix until crumbly dough forms. Press the mixture into a casserole dish & bake at 350 F for 20 to 25 minutes.

4. Remove; set aside and let completely cool at room temperature, then refrigerate for an hour. Cut into slices; serve and enjoy.

BLACKBERRY COCONUT FAT BOMBS

Prep Time: 10 minutes
Cooking Time: 5 minutes
Servings: 16

Nutritional Info (Estimated Amount Per Serving)

- 230 Calories

- 215 Calories from Fat

- 24g Total Fat

- 20g Saturated Fat

- 0g Trans Fat

- 0.4g Polyunsaturated Fat

- 1.3g Monounsaturated Fat

- 0mg Cholesterol

- 6.2mg Sodium

- 95mg Potassium

- 4.4g Total Carbohydrates

- 2.9g Dietary Fiber

- 1.4g Sugars

- 1.2g Protein

INGREDIENTS

- ½ cup blackberries (can be substituted with strawberries or raspberries), fresh or frozen

- 1 cup coconut oil

- ½ tsp. stevia drops or to taste

- 1 tbsp. lemon juice, fresh

- ½ tsp. vanilla extract or ¼ tsp. vanilla powder

- 1 cup coconut butter, homemade

DIRECTIONS

1. Place blackberries together with, coconut butter and coconut oil over medium heat settings in a large pot; heat until combined well.

2. Add coconut oil mixture & the leftover ingredients together in a blender or food processor; process on high settings until smooth.

3. Spread the mixture out into a 6x6" container.

4. Refrigerate until the mixture has hardened, for an hour.

5. Carefully remove from the container & then cut into squares.

6. Cover and store in the refrigerator until ready to serve.

ENGLISH TOFFEE FAT BOMBS

Prep Time: 10 minutes
Cooking Time: 2 hours & 20 minutes
Servings: 6

Nutritional Info (Estimated Amount Per Serving)

- 636 Calories

- 540 Calories from Fat

- 60g Total Fat

- 39g Saturated Fat

- 0.2g Trans Fat

- 3.4g Polyunsaturated Fat

- 12g Monounsaturated Fat

- 37mg Cholesterol

- 187mg Sodium

- 174mg Potassium

- 20g Total Carbohydrates

- 2g Dietary Fiber

- 12g Sugars

- 6.9g Protein

INGREDIENTS

- 4 oz. cream cheese

- ¾ tbsp. cocoa powder

- 3 tbsp. English toffee syrup, sugar-free

- 1 cup coconut oil

- ½ cup natural peanut butter

- 2 tbsp. butter

DIRECTIONS

1. Put the entire ingredients together over medium-low heat settings in a large pot. Give everything a good stir until completely smooth and melted.

2. Pour the mixture into a mini muffin pan or silicone pans mold. Place the pan in a freezer and let freeze for a couple of hours, until set.

3. Once done, carefully remove them from the molds. Serve immediately and enjoy or store them in an air-tight container in the freezer.

LEMON-CURD
FAT BOMB

Prep Time: 10 minutes
Cooking Time: 20 minutes
Servings: 24

Nutritional Info (Estimated Amount Per Serving)

- 98 Calories

- 90 Calories from Fat

- 10g Total Fat

- 6.8g Saturated Fat

- 0g Trans Fat

- 0.4g Polyunsaturated Fat

- 2.1g Monounsaturated Fat

- 31mg Cholesterol

- 43mg Sodium

- 18mg Potassium

- 1.2g Total Carbohydrates

- 0.1g Dietary Fiber

- 0.2g Sugars

- 1.1g Protein

INGREDIENTS

For Filling:

- 1 tbsp. lemon peel, finely grated
- ½ cup lemon juice, fresh
- 8 tbsp. coconut oil
- 1 cup erythritol or Swerve
- 4 eggs, large

For Coating:

- 1 tsp. lemon extract
- ⅔ cup Swerve confectioners
- 4 oz. edible cocoa butter
- ¼ tsp. Celtic sea salt

DIRECTIONS

1. Heat the cocoa butter over medium-high heat settings in a double boiler until completely melted

2. Once done; add in the natural sweetener together with extracts & salt; don't forget to stir everything together after each addition.

3. Place the mixture into truffle mold & let cool in a refrigerator for an hour, until completely set.

For Lemon Curd Filling:

1. Combine lemon juice together with lemon peel, natural sweetener and 4 eggs over medium heat settings in a medium, heavy saucepan. Whisk until completely blended; add in the coconut oil. Continue to whisk for 10 to 12 minutes, until the mixture

thickens (don't bring it to a boil). Transfer the mixture through a strainer into a medium-sized bowl. Now, fill a large bowl (large enough to cover the bowl) with ice water and then place the bowl with the mixture in it; whisk every now and then for 12 to 15 minutes, until lemon curd is completely cooled.

To Make Truffle:

1. It's time to remove the molds from freezer or fridge & fill them with the lemon curd filling. Once done; top the filling with a layer of the cocoa butter. Place the mold into freezer/fridge again until set.

FUDGY MACADAMIA CHOCOLATE FAT BOMBS

Prep Time: 5 minutes
Cooking Time: 35 minutes
Servings: 6

Nutritional Info (Estimated Amount Per Serving)

- 307 Calories

- 296 Calories from Fat

- 33g Total Fat

- 15g Saturated Fat

- 0g Trans Fat

- 0.7g Polyunsaturated Fat

- 15g Monounsaturated Fat

- 0mg Cholesterol

- 1mg Sodium

- 70mg Potassium

- 3.6g Total Carbohydrates

- 2g Dietary Fiber

- 0.9g Sugars

- 1.8g Protein

INGREDIENTS

- 2 tbsp. Swerve

- 4 oz. macadamias, chopped

- 2 oz. cocoa butter

- ¼ cup coconut oil or heavy cream

- 2 tbsp. cocoa powder, unsweetened

DIRECTIONS

1. Melt the cocoa butter in a bath of water in a small-sized sauce pan.

2. Once done; add in the cocoa powder followed by the Swerve; mix well until completely melted and blended well.

3. Stir in the macadamias.

4. Now, add the cream; mix well & bring it to the heat again.

5. Pour the prepared mixture in the molds.

6. Set aside and let cool completely, then place it inside the fridge until harden, for an hour. Serve immediately and enjoy.

MATCHA COCONUT FAT BOMBS

Prep Time: 5 minutes
Cooking Time: 55 minutes
Servings: 32

Nutritional Info (Estimated Amount Per Serving)

- 138 Calories

- 129 Calories from Fat

- 14g Total Fat

- 12g Saturated Fat

- 0g Trans Fat

- 0.2g Polyunsaturated Fat

- 0.8g Monounsaturated Fat

- 0mg Cholesterol

- 17mg Sodium

- 66mg Potassium

- 2.7g Total Carbohydrates

- 1.7g Dietary Fiber

- 0.8g Sugars

- 0.8g Protein

INGREDIENTS

For The Truffles:

- ½ cup full fat coconut milk, refrigerated for overnight

- 1 tsp. pure vanilla extract

- ¼ tsp. ground Ceylon cinnamon

- 1 cup creamy coconut butter

- ½ tsp. matcha green tea powder

- 1 cup firm coconut oil

- ¼ tsp. Himalayan salt

For The Coating

- 1 tbsp. Matcha green tea powder

- 1 cup unsweetened coconut, finely shredded

DIRECTIONS

1. Add the entire truffles ingredients together to a large-sized mixing bowl.

2. Using a hand mixer; mix until light & fluffy, for a couple of minutes, on high speed. Place in a refrigerator for an hour, until set.

3. In the meantime; in a fairly large mixing bowl, combine shredded coconut together with the matcha powder; mix well and set aside.

4. Form approximately 32 ping-pong sized balls from the cold "truffle" mixture using a small-sized ice cream scoop.

5. Roll the balls immediately between the palms of your hands and

then drop all the balls into the matcha-coconut mixture; rolling them into the mixture until coated completely.

6. Transfer the coated fat bombs into an air-tight container; keep refrigerated until ready to serve.

RASPBERRY ALMOND CHOCOLATE FAT BOMBS

Prep Time: 5 minutes
Cooking Time: 1 hour & 10 minutes
Servings: 8

Nutritional Info (Estimated Amount Per Serving)

- 190 Calories
- 159 Calories from Fat
- 18g Total Fat
- 9.7g Saturated Fat
- 0g Trans Fat
- 2.7g Polyunsaturated Fat
- 4g Monounsaturated Fat
- 0mg Cholesterol
- 6.6mg Sodium
- 184mg Potassium
- 7.4g Total Carbohydrates
- 4.4g Dietary Fiber
- 2g Sugars
- 3.8g Protein

INGREDIENTS

- ¼ tsp. stevia powder

- 1 tbsp. cocoa powder, unsweetened

- ¼ cup frozen raspberries

- 20 g almonds, raw, chopped

- ½ cup coconut butter

- 20 g walnuts, chopped

- ¼ cup almond butter

DIRECTIONS

1. Mix the almond butter together with coconut butter, cocoa powder and stevia powder in a large bowl.

2. Place the raspberries in a large bowl and microwave for half a minute to a minute.

3. Place few parchment papers on top of a square pan & then add the chocolate butter. Sprinkle with the chopped nuts & then cover them with the heated & melted raspberries. Set aside and let cool until easy to handle.

4. Now, place in the freezer until set, for an hour. Remove & break it into eight even-sized pieces. Serve and enjoy.

WHITE CHOCOLATE PECAN BUTTER FAT BOMBS

Prep Time: 15 minutes
Cooking Time: 20 minutes
Servings: 8

Nutritional Info (Estimated Amount Per Serving)

- 188 Calories

- 185 Calories from Fat

- 21g Total Fat

- 8.7g Saturated Fat

- 0g Trans Fat

- 2.5g Polyunsaturated Fat

- 8.3g Monounsaturated Fat

- 7.6mg Cholesterol

- 17mg Sodium

- 41mg Potassium

- 7.1g Total Carbohydrates

- 0.9g Dietary Fiber

- 0.4g Sugars

- 0.9g Protein

INGREDIENTS

- 1 oz. unsalted butter

- ½ teaspoon pure vanilla extract

- 15 to 20 drops of liquid stevia or to taste

- ¾ cup walnuts or pecans, chopped & toasted

- 3 oz. cacao butter

- A pinch of sea salt

DIRECTIONS

1. Over moderate heat settings in a large pan; heat the unsalted butter together with cacao butter until completely melted and then add the salt, stevia, pecans, and vanilla; don't forget to give everything a good stir after each addition.

2. Spoon the mixture evenly into eight silicone muffin wells.

3. Transfer to the fridge and let chill for an hour, until set.

4. Serve and enjoy. Feel free to store the leftovers in the fridge in an air-tight container for up to 3 weeks.

EASTER EGG
FAT BOMBS

Prep Time: 35 minutes
Cooking Time: 20 minutes
Servings: 14

Nutritional Info (Estimated Amount Per Serving)

- 249 Calories

- 213 Calories from Fat

- 24g Total Fat

- 13g Saturated Fat

- 0g Trans Fat

- 2.2g Polyunsaturated Fat

- 6.4g Monounsaturated Fat

- 0mg Cholesterol

- 41mg Sodium

- 167mg Potassium

- 9.5g Total Carbohydrates

- 3.9g Dietary Fiber

- 1.4g Sugars

- 4.5g Protein

INGREDIENTS

- 5-10 drops of stevia, alcohol-free

- ½ cup coconut oil, melted

- 2 cups Almond Flour

- ⅓ cup sugar-free dark chocolate chips

- 1 teaspoon vanilla extract, alcohol-free

- ¼ teaspoon gray sea salt

For Coating:

- Natural food coloring, preferably Easter-themed

- ½ cup melted coconut butter

DIRECTIONS

1. Lay silicon baking mat or a parchment paper over a baking sheet, preferably large-sized.

2. Add vanilla together with almond flour, stevia, coconut oil & salt to a food processor. Process on high settings for several seconds, until completely smooth.

3. Fold in the chocolate chips & scoop approximately 1 ½ tbsp. of the mixture; roll into a ball using your palms. Now, place the prepared balls over the prepared baking sheet; flatten & shaping into a large egg. Repeat these steps with the leftover dough.

4. Transfer the baking sheet to a freezer & let chill for an hour.

5. Place a cooling rack on top of a second baking sheet; set aside.

6. For frosting: Over moderate heat settings in a large pan; heat the coconut butter until melted, evenly divide the melted butter into separate dishes & then add in the food coloring.

7. Remove the cookie dough eggs from freezer. Dip first side of each into the coconut butter & place them over the cooling rack. Add the leftover colored coconut butter to a large-sized Ziploc bag; cut the tip out & drizzle on top.

8. Transfer the eggs over cooling rack into a fridge and let chill for an hour, until set. Serve and enjoy.

ALMOND BUTTER CHIA SEEDS FAT BOMBS

Prep Time: 10 minutes
Cooking Time: 3 hours & 30 minutes
Servings: 8

Nutritional Info (Estimated Amount Per Serving)

- 240 Calories

- 169 Calories from Fat

- 19g Total Fat

- 11g Saturated Fat

- 0.2g Trans Fat

- 2.6g Polyunsaturated Fat

- 4.1g Monounsaturated Fat

- 16mg Cholesterol

- 39mg Sodium

- 140mg Potassium

- 16g Total Carbohydrates

- 4.1g Dietary Fiber

- 11g Sugars

- 3.4g Protein

INGREDIENTS

- ¼ cup chia seeds

- 1 tbsp. plus 1 tsp. coconut oil

- ¼ cup heavy whipping cream

- 2 tbsp. butter

- ½ cup unsweetened coconut flakes, shredded

- 1 ½ tsp. vanilla extract

- ¼ tsp. liquid Stevia

- 4 tbsp. erythritol

- ½ cup coconut cream

- 2 tbsp. coconut flour

- ½ cup almonds, raw

DIRECTIONS

1. Place the toasted almonds in a food processor & grind until mealy substance forms. Add 2 tbsp. of erythritol & 1 tsp. of coconut oil; continue to mix until you get almond butter.

2. Now, over moderate heat settings in a pan; heat the butter until melted & turns browned. Now, add heavy cream together with stevia, vanilla, and 2 tbsp. erythritol; continue to mix until you get bubbly mixture like consistency. Transfer almond butter to the mixture; give everything a good stir until evenly mixed.

3. In the meantime, using a spice grinder; grind the chia seeds. Now, toast the coconut flakes and chia seeds together in a pan for a couple of minutes.

4. Add in the coconut cream, coconut flour, and 1 tbsp. coconut

oil & combine everything together. Mix well & place the mixture into a square dish.

5. Place the dish in a refrigerator and let chill for an hour, until set. Once done; chop into small even-sized squares & place them in a refrigerator again for a couple of hours. Serve and enjoy.

MOUTHWATERING COCONUT FAT BOMBS

Prep Time: 15 minutes
Cooking Time: 55 minutes
Servings: 12

Nutritional Info (Estimated Amount Per Serving)

- 130 Calories

- 108 Calories from Fat

- 12g Total Fat

- 10g Saturated Fat

- 0g Trans Fat

- 0.2g Polyunsaturated Fat

- 0.7g Monounsaturated Fat

- 0mg Cholesterol

- 38mg Sodium

- 38mg Potassium

- 13g Total Carbohydrates

- 1.1g Dietary Fiber

- 3.9g Sugars

- 0.3g Protein

INGREDIENTS

- ¼ tsp vanilla bean powder or cinnamon

- 1 ½ cup unsweetened flaked coconut or shredded, desiccated coconut

- ¼ cup extra virgin coconut oil

- 20 to 25 drops of Stevia extract

- ¼ cup grass-fed butter (chopped into pieces) or coconut oil

- A pinch of Himalayan pink salt

DIRECTIONS

1. Preheat your oven to 350 F in advance. Spread the flaked or shredded coconut on a large-sized baking sheet and then place the sheet in the preheated oven. Toast until turns light golden, for 5 to 8 minutes. To prevent burning; don't forget to mix the coconut a couple of times. Transfer the toasted coconut to a blender; pulse on high settings until smooth.

2. Add softened coconut oil and softened butter and then add vanilla or cinnamon, stevia, and salt; don't forget to give everything a good stir after each addition.

3. Pour the mixture into an ice cube tray or mini muffin forms. Place in a fridge and let chill until solidify, for half an hour.

4. When done, serve immediately and enjoy!

CHOCOLATE HEMP FAT BOMB

Prep Time: 5 minutes
Cooking Time: 1 hour & 10 minutes
Servings: 6

Nutritional Info (Estimated Amount Per Serving)

- 119 Calories
- 106 Calories from Fat
- 12g Total Fat
- 9.6g Saturated Fat
- 0g Trans Fat
- 0.6g Polyunsaturated Fat
- 0.7g Monounsaturated Fat
- 0mg Cholesterol
- 52mg Sodium
- 33mg Potassium
- 1.7g Total Carbohydrates
- 0.6g Dietary Fiber
- 0.3g Sugars
- 3g Protein

INGREDIENTS

- ¼ cup extra-virgin coconut oil, melted

- 2 drop of liquid stevia, alcohol-free

- ¼ cup coconut, unsweetened, toasted

- A pinch of Himalayan rock salt

- 3 tablespoons Harvest Chocolate Hemp Protein Powder

- ¼ tsp vanilla extract, alcohol-free

DIRECTIONS

1. Spread the unsweetened coconut on a baking sheet, preferably small-sized. Preheat your oven to 325 F in advance. Place the baking sheet with the coconut in the preheated oven & roast for a couple of minutes. Don't let it burn.

2. Add Chocolate Hemp Protein Powder to a bowl, preferably small-sized. Add in the leftover ingredients; give everything a good stir until the mixture is evenly mixed.

3. Evenly divide the mixture into a silicone candy mold. Place in a fridge and let chill for an hour, until set.

4. Serve and enjoy!

CHOCONUT ALMOND BUTTER FAT BOMBS

Prep Time: 15 minutes
Cooking Time: 20 minutes
Servings: 12

Nutritional Info (Estimated Amount Per Serving)

- 312 Calories

- 258 Calories from Fat

- 29g Total Fat

- 20g Saturated Fat

- 0g Trans Fat

- 1.8g Polyunsaturated Fat

- 4.7g Monounsaturated Fat

- 0mg Cholesterol

- 25mg Sodium

- 165mg Potassium

- 11g Total Carbohydrates

- 4.5g Dietary Fiber

- 4g Sugars

- 4.1g Protein

INGREDIENTS

For Bottom Layer:

- ¼ tsp ground Ceylon cinnamon

- 1 tsp vanilla powder

- ½ cup cacao paste, chopped finely

- 2-3 drops of almond extract, pure

- ¼ cup coconut oil

For Second Layer:

- ¼ cup coconut oil

- ½ cup natural almond butter

- ¼ tsp ground Ceylon cinnamon

For Final Layer:

- ½ cup creamy coconut butter

- ¼ cup coconut oil

For Garnish:

- Coconut flakes, toasted

- Whole almonds, raw

DIRECTIONS

1. Line a standard sized muffin pan with silicone cups or parchment lined paper cups, preferably large-sized.

2. Now, heat approximately ¾ cup of the coconut oil over moderate heat settings in a large pan until completely melted.

3. Now, heat the cacao paste in the microwave until completely melted in a small-sized mixing bowl (work in 20 to 30 seconds intervals); stir well until no lumps remain; stir in approximately ¼ cup of heated coconut oil, cinnamon, almond extract and vanilla powder. Continue to mix until combined completely.

4. Evenly distribute the heated chocolate among the muffin cups & place the tin in a fridge for a couple of minutes, until set.

5. In the meantime, add almond butter together with ¼ cup of melted coconut oil and ground cinnamon in a separate mixing bowl. Continue to stir until evenly combined and then pour the mixture on top of the firmed up chocolate. Place the cups into the fridge again for a couple of more minutes, until this layer firms up as well.

6. In the meantime, add approximately half a cup of the coconut butter into the melted coconut oil; give everything a good stir until incorporated well.

7. Spoon the mixture delicately over the layer of almond butter and then garnish every cup with a pinch of coconut flakes (toasted) or a whole almond.

8. Place the cups again into the refrigerator and let chill for an hour, until set. Serve immediately and enjoy or store them in an air-tight container in the refrigerator.

ORANGE & WALNUT CHOCOLATE FAT BOMBS

Prep Time: 15 minutes
Cooking Time: 2 hours & 20 minutes
Servings: 25

Nutritional Info (Estimated Amount Per Serving)

- 56 Calories

- 52 Calories from Fat

- 5.8g Total Fat

- 2.1g Saturated Fat

- 0g Trans Fat

- 2.7g Polyunsaturated Fat

- 0.6g Monounsaturated Fat

- 0mg Cholesterol

- 0.2mg Sodium

- 26mg Potassium

- 2.3g Total Carbohydrates

- 0.4g Dietary Fiber

- 0.2g Sugars

- 0.9g Protein

INGREDIENTS

- 4.4 oz 85% to 90% dark cocoa chocolate

- 10 to 15 drops of liquid Stevia

- ½ to 1 tbsp. orange extract, sugar-free or orange zest, fresh

- 1 1/3 cup walnuts, roughly chopped

- 1 tsp. cinnamon

- ¼ cup extra virgin coconut oil

DIRECTIONS

1. Melt the dark chocolate in a large bowl in a water bath (ensure the bowl don't touch the water). Add coconut oil together with cinnamon, and stevia; mix well.

2. Now, add in the orange food extract and fresh orange peel.

3. Add walnuts; mix well again.

4. Evenly spoon the mixture into candy cups or paper muffin, small-sized.

5. Place in a fridge and let chill until set, for a few hours. Serve and enjoy.

DARK CHOCOLATE & NUT FAT BOMBS

Prep Time: 10 minutes
Cooking Time: 40 minutes
Servings: 16

Nutritional Info (Estimated Amount Per Serving)

- 50 Calories

- 47 Calories from Fat

- 5.3g Total Fat

- 4.4g Saturated Fat

- 0g Trans Fat

- 0.1g Polyunsaturated Fat

- 0.3g Monounsaturated Fat

- 0mg Cholesterol

- 1.4mg Sodium

- 1.3mg Potassium

- 3.1g Total Carbohydrates

- 0g Dietary Fiber

- 0.1g Sugars

- 0g Protein

INGREDIENTS

- 1 oz. extra virgin coconut oil or cocoa butter

- 2 oz. coconut oil, ghee or butter

- 1 tbsp. unsweetened vanilla extract or 1 tsp. vanilla powder

- 4 oz. 85% dark cacao chocolate

- 2 tbsp. Swerve or Erythritol, powdered

- 10 to 20 drops of liquid Stevia extract

- 1/3 cup nut butter

DIRECTIONS

1. Over medium-heat settings in a double boiler; melt the cacao butter together with dark chocolate. Once done, turn the heat off.

2. Add in the macadamia butter, vanilla powder, and powdered Erythritol; mix until combined well. Add in the butter; give everything a good stir until evenly mixed. Pour approximately 2 tbsp. of chocolate mixture into an ice cube tray or mini muffin forms.

3. Place the tray inside the fridge until solidify, for half an hour. Serve immediately and enjoy or store them in an air-tight container in a refrigerator until ready to serve.

COCONUT CINNAMON FAT BOMBS

Prep Time: 15 minutes
Cooking Time: 55 minutes
Servings: 10

Nutritional Info (Estimated Amount Per Serving)

- 254 Calories

- 214 Calories from Fat

- 24g Total Fat

- 21g Saturated Fat

- 0g Trans Fat

- 0.3g Polyunsaturated Fat

- 1g Monounsaturated Fat

- 0mg Cholesterol

- 37mg Sodium

- 221mg Potassium

- 12g Total Carbohydrates

- 5.1g Dietary Fiber

- 5.1g Sugars

- 2.5g Protein

INGREDIENTS

- 1 cup full-fat coconut milk, canned

- 1 cup coconut butter

- 1 tsp. stevia powder extract

- ½ tsp. nutmeg

- 1 cup coconut shreds

- ½ tsp. cinnamon

- 1 tsp. vanilla extract

DIRECTIONS

1. In a large bowl; place the entire ingredients (don't add the shredded coconut) over medium heat settings in a double boiler.

2. Mix well and let melt (continue to mix).

3. When done; remove the bowl immediately from heat. Set aside and let cool at room temperature until easy to handle.

4. Place the bowl in the fridge and let chill for half an hour, until you can easily form balls from the mixture.

5. Form ping-pong sized balls from the mixture; rolling each bowl through the coconut shreds.

6. Now, arrange the coated balls on a clean, large plate & let refrigerate for an hour again.

PEPPERMINT FAT BOMBS

Prep Time: 5 minutes
Cooking Time: 1 hour & 10 minutes
Servings: 6

Nutritional Info (Estimated Amount Per Serving)

- 251 Calories

- 244 Calories from Fat

- 27g Total Fat

- 22g Saturated Fat

- 0g Trans Fat

- 0.5g Polyunsaturated Fat

- 1.7g Monounsaturated Fat

- 0mg Cholesterol

- 0mg Sodium

- 0.1mg Potassium

- 1.2g Total Carbohydrates

- 0.3g Dietary Fiber

- 0.2g Sugars

- 0.3g Protein

INGREDIENTS

- 2 tbsp. unsweetened cocoa

- ¼ tsp. peppermint essence

- 1 tbsp. granulated sweetener or to taste

- ¾ cup melted coconut oil

DIRECTIONS

1. Thoroughly combine the melted coconut oil together with peppermint essence and sweetener of your choice.

2. Pour ½ of the prepared mixture into ice cube trays or silicon cases. Place the trays inside the fridge and let chill until you can see a white layer on the top.

3. Now, add cocoa powder to the leftover mixture and then pour the mixture over white layer.

4. Place the trays into the fridge again and let chill until completely set.

CHOCONUT ALMOND BUTTER FAT BOMBS

Prep Time: 15 minutes
Cooking Time: 20 minutes
Servings: 8

Nutritional Info (Estimated Amount Per Serving)

- 129 Calories
- 113 Calories from Fat
- 13g Total Fat
- 6.7g Saturated Fat
- 0.2g Trans Fat
- 0.9g Polyunsaturated Fat
- 3.8g Monounsaturated Fat
- 31mg Cholesterol
- 64mg Sodium
- 62mg Potassium
- 2.9g Total Carbohydrates
- 0.4g Dietary Fiber
- 1.5g Sugars
- 2.4g Protein

INGREDIENTS

- ½ square chocolate shavings, unsweetened, grated

- 4 oz. cream cheese

- ½ cup heavy whipping cream

- 3-4 packets of stevia

- ½ tsp. vanilla

- 2 tbsp. Natural peanut butter

DIRECTIONS

1. Add heavy whipping cream in a medium-sized mixing bowl; whip until stiff peaks form; set aside.

2. Add peanut butter together with cream cheese, stevia, and vanilla in a separate bowl; mix until smooth, preferably on medium speed.

3. Add cream cheese mixture to the whipped cream; continue to mix until fluffy, on medium speed.

4. Add the grated chocolate shavings over the top.

5. Refrigerator for overnight. Serve chilled and enjoy.

STRAWBERRY FAT BOMBS

Prep Time: 15 minutes
Cooking Time: 2 hours & 20 minutes
Servings: 12

Nutritional Info (Estimated Amount Per Serving)

- 109 Calories

- 91 Calories from Fat

- 10g Total Fat

- 7.3g Saturated Fat

- 0.2g Trans Fat

- 0.3g Polyunsaturated Fat

- 1.7g Monounsaturated Fat

- 16mg Cholesterol

- 32mg Sodium

- 13mg Potassium

- 4.7g Total Carbohydrates

- 0.1g Dietary Fiber

- 4.5g Sugars

- 0.2g Protein

INGREDIENTS

- 3 regular-sized strawberries, diced (approximately 50 grams)

- 4 tbsp. butter

- 1 tbsp. plus 2 tsp. Truvia or ¼ cup sugar

- 2 ounces heavy cream

- 4 tbsp. coconut oil

DIRECTIONS

1. Add heavy cream to the diced strawberries in a large bowl and then blend them together using an immersion blender.

2. Now, heat the butter for half a minute in the microwave; set aside.

3. Measure the coconut oil out & set aside; don't heat the oil.

4. Add in the sweetener & combine everything together using an immersion blender.

5. Now, spoon the mixture or pipe it into the mold using a piping bag.

6. Place the molds into a freezer and let chill until set, for half an hour.

7. Once set; carefully remove the fat-bombs from the mold and arrange them on a wax paper. Melt a piece of sugar-free chocolate in advance.

8. For a real peep look; dab on nose and eyes with a toothpick. Place them to the freezer again and let chill for 10 to 20 more minutes. Serve immediately and enjoy.

CHOCOLATE RASPBERRY FAT BOMBS

Prep Time: 10 minutes
Cooking Time: 2 hours & 10 minutes
Servings: 6

Nutritional Info (Estimated Amount Per Serving)

- 191 Calories

- 149 Calories from Fat

- 17g Total Fat

- 12g Saturated Fat

- 0.4g Trans Fat

- 0.5g Polyunsaturated Fat

- 2.9g Monounsaturated Fat

- 25mg Cholesterol

- 85mg Sodium

- 8.1mg Potassium

- 11g Total Carbohydrates

- 0.5g Dietary Fiber

- 5.9g Sugars

- 0.5g Protein

INGREDIENTS

- 2 tbsp. raspberry syrup, sugar-free

- 5 tbsp. butter

- 2 tbsp. cocoa powder

- 3 tbsp. coconut oil

DIRECTIONS

1. Over very low-heat settings in a large sauce pan; combine the entire ingredients together until you get a consistency of chocolate sauce.

2. Pour the mixture into mold & freeze for a couple of hours in a refrigerator, until set.

3. Once done; carefully remove them from the molds; serve and enjoy.

BLACK & WHITE PEPPERMINT BOMBS

Prep Time: 15 minutes
Cooking Time: 55 minutes
Servings: 12

Nutritional Info (Estimated Amount Per Serving)

- 148 Calories

- 129 Calories from Fat

- 14g Total Fat

- 13g Saturated Fat

- 0g Trans Fat

- 0.2g Polyunsaturated Fat

- 0.7g Monounsaturated Fat

- 0mg Cholesterol

- 13mg Sodium

- 96mg Potassium

- 9g Total Carbohydrates

- 2.9g Dietary Fiber

- 2.1g Sugars

- 1.2g Protein

INGREDIENTS

- 1/3 cup shredded coconut

- 2 tsp. cocoa powder, unsweetened

- ½ tsp. peppermint extract

- 3 tbsp. coconut oil

- ¾ cup coconut butter

- 15 to 20 drops of liquid stevia or to taste

DIRECTIONS

1. Combine shredded coconut together with coconut butter, peppermint extract, and 1 tbsp. coconut oil in a large bowl using an immerse blender. Mix well & pour the mixture into mini muffin tins or cupcake liners or molds.

2. Place the molds into the fridge and let chill for several minutes, until solidify.

3. Mix the leftover coconut oil with cocoa powder; mix well. Once the molds are set; remove from the refrigerator & pour the prepared cocoa mixture over the top. Place it in the fridge again and let chill for a couple of more minutes, until firm.

4. Serve and enjoy.

BLACKBERRY NUT FAT BOMBS

Prep Time: 5 minutes
Cooking Time: 1 hour & 10 minutes
Servings: 12

Nutritional Info (Estimated Amount Per Serving)

- 406 Calories

- 377 Calories from Fat

- 42g Total Fat

- 32g Saturated Fat

- 0.1g Trans Fat

- 0.8g Polyunsaturated Fat

- 6.2g Monounsaturated Fat

- 19mg Cholesterol

- 68mg Sodium

- 173mg Potassium

- 7.9g Total Carbohydrates

- 4.5g Dietary Fiber

- 2.9g Sugars

- 2.9g Protein

INGREDIENTS

- 1 cup blackberries, fresh

- 4 oz. cream cheese or neufchatel cheese

- 1 cup coconut butter

- 2 oz. crushed macadamia nuts

- ½ tsp. vanilla extract

- 3 tbsp. mascarpone cheese

- Stevia to taste

- 1 cup coconut oil

- ½ tsp. lemon juice

DIRECTIONS

1. Press the crushed macadamia nuts into the bottom of a mold or baking dish. Bake at 325 F until turn golden brown, for 5 to 7 minutes.

2. Remove the nuts from oven; set aside at room temperature and let slightly cool until easy to handle.

3. Now, spread a layer of the softened cream cheese on top of the nut crust.

4. Thoroughly combine the blackberries together with coconut butter, vanilla, coconut oil, mascarpone cheese, sweetener and lemon juice in a large bowl until smooth, for a couple of minutes.

5. Pour the mixture on top of the cream cheese layer. Freeze until set, for half an hour to an hour. Serve immediately and enjoy.

BLUEBERRY COCONUT CREAM FAT BOMBS

Prep Time: 15 minutes
Cooking Time: 2 hours & 20 minutes
Servings: 16

Nutritional Info (Estimated Amount Per Serving)

- 233 Calories

- 216 Calories from Fat

- 24g Total Fat

- 17g Saturated Fat

- 0g Trans Fat

- 0.7g Polyunsaturated Fat

- 4.4g Monounsaturated Fat

- 36mg Cholesterol

- 27mg Sodium

- 26mg Potassium

- 4.2g Total Carbohydrates

- 0.2g Dietary Fiber

- 3.5g Sugars

- 0.9g Protein

INGREDIENTS

- 4 oz. softened neufchatel cheese

- 1 cup blueberries, fresh, crushed

- ¼ cup coconut cream

- 8 oz. butter, unsalted

- Liquid stevia to taste

- ¾ cup coconut oil

DIRECTIONS

1. Place the blueberries in the bottom of a pan or dish. Now, over low-heat settings in a large saucepan; heat the coconut oil with butter until melted. Once done; immediately remove the pan from heat; set aside and let cool for a couple of minutes.

2. Now, add the leftover ingredients; whip well with a hand blender or whisk, slowly adding the stevia.

3. Pour the prepared mixture into the saucepan & place in a freezer; let chill for an hour. Just before serving; slice into pieces and top each piece with some whole blueberries.

TOASTED COCONUT FAT BOMB BARK

Prep Time: 15 minutes
Cooking Time: 2 hours & 20 minutes
Servings: 6

Nutritional Info (Estimated Amount Per Serving)

- 421 Calories

- 389 Calories from Fat

- 43g Total Fat

- 32g Saturated Fat

- 0g Trans Fat

- 1.1g Polyunsaturated Fat

- 7.1g Monounsaturated Fat

- 31mg Cholesterol

- 110mg Sodium

- 131mg Potassium

- 14g Total Carbohydrates

- 2.9g Dietary Fiber

- 1.1g Sugars

- 2.5g Protein

INGREDIENTS

- 3 oz. baking chocolate, unsweetened
- 15 to 20 drops of liquid stevia or to taste
- 3 tbsp. large coconut flakes, unsweetened
- 1 ½ tbsp. cocoa powder
- 5 oz. coconut oil
- 3 oz. unsalted butter
- ¼ tsp. salt

DIRECTIONS

1. Preheat your oven to 350 F in advance. Place the large flaked unsweetened coconut on a baking sheet and toast in the preheated oven, checking every now and then (don't let it burn).

2. Now, over medium heat settings in a microwave; heat the coconut oil together with unsalted butter and unsweetened dark chocolate for a couple of minutes, until melted.

3. Add in the cocoa powder, stevia & salt; give everything a good stir until evenly mixed.

4. Place a small quantity of toasted coconut in every section of mold or silicone ice cube tray and then pour the chocolate mixture over the top. Sprinkle more coconut flakes over the top, if desired. Place the molds into the fridge and let chill until hardened, for an hour. Serve and enjoy.

STUFFED PECAN
FAT BOMBS

Prep Time: 10 minutes
Cooking Time: 40 minutes
Servings: 1

Nutritional Info (Estimated Amount Per Serving)

- 158 Calories

- 142 Calories from Fat

- 16g Total Fat

- 7.6g Saturated Fat

- 0g Trans Fat

- 1.7g Polyunsaturated Fat

- 5g Monounsaturated Fat

- 29mg Cholesterol

- 222mg Sodium

- 76mg Potassium

- 6.5g Total Carbohydrates

- 1g Dietary Fiber

- 1.5g Sugars

- 2.5g Protein

INGREDIENTS

- 4 pecan halves

- 1 oz. cream cheese or neufchatel cheese

- ½ tsp. coconut butter or unsalted butter

- Stevia to taste

- A pinch of sea salt

DIRECTIONS

1. Preheat your oven to 350 F in advance. Place the pecans in a baking sheet and toast in the preheated oven for a couple of minutes; set aside & let cool until easy to handle.

2. Soften the cream cheese and butter, add in the remaining ingredients (except salt); mix until smooth & creamy.

3. Now, spread the cream cheese-butter mix between 2 pecan halves and sprinkle a small pinch of sea salt over the top. Serve immediately and enjoy.

STRAWBERRY MOCHA SWIRL FAT BOMBS

Prep Time: 15 minutes
Cooking Time: 55 minutes
Servings: 12

Nutritional Info (Estimated Amount Per Serving)

- 104 Calories

- 99 Calories from Fat

- 11g Total Fat

- 8g Saturated Fat

- 0g Trans Fat

- 0.3g Polyunsaturated Fat

- 1.9g Monounsaturated Fat

- 14mg Cholesterol

- 1.1mg Sodium

- 20mg Potassium

- 1.5g Total Carbohydrates

- 0.4g Dietary Fiber

- 0.6g Sugars

- 0.3g Protein

INGREDIENTS

- 2 tbsp. cocoa powder

- 4 tbsp. coconut oil

- ¼ tsp. liquid stevia or to taste

- 4 tbsp. unsalted butter

For Strawberry Swirl:

- 1 tbsp. heavy cream

- ¼ cup strawberries, fresh, mashed

- 1 tbsp. unsalted butter

- ¼ tsp. of liquid stevia

- 1 tbsp. coconut oil

DIRECTIONS

1. Soften the butter in a microwave; set aside at room temperature and let slightly cool. Now, to the melted butter; add cocoa powder together with coconut oil, and stevia; mix well using a hand blender; set aside until ready to use.

For Strawberry Swirl:

1. Add heavy cream to the mashed strawberries & microwave until warm, for a couple of minutes; set aside.

2. Now, over melt the butter & add it together with stevia and coconut oil to the strawberry mix. Whisk rapidly or mix well using a stick blender.

For Assembling:

1. Pour the prepared chocolate mixture into cupcake liners or mold. Add strawberry to the middle & swirl with a clean toothpick.

2. Place the liners or mold into a freezer and let chill for several minutes, then carefully remove the fat bombs from the mold. Serve and enjoy.

VANILLA COCONUT FAT BOMBS

Prep Time: 5 minutes
Cooking Time: 1 hour & 10 minutes
Servings: 6

Nutritional Info (Estimated Amount Per Serving)

- 135 Calories
- 123 Calories from Fat
- 14g Total Fat
- 12g Saturated Fat
- 0g Trans Fat
- 0.2g Polyunsaturated Fat
- 0.7g Monounsaturated Fat
- 0mg Cholesterol
- 52mg Sodium
- 77mg Potassium
- 3.8g Total Carbohydrates
- 2.3g Dietary Fiber
- 1.1g Sugars
- 1g Protein

INGREDIENTS

- 1 cup shredded coconut, unsweetened

- ½ tsp. vanilla extract

- 2 tbsp. coconut oil (or MCT oil)

- ¼ cup water

- Liquid stevia to taste

- 1/8 tsp. salt

DIRECTIONS

1. Combine the entire ingredients together in a food processor; process on high settings until smooth and creamy. Pour the mixture into molds.

2. Place the molds into a refrigerator and let chill until set, for an hour. Serve and enjoy.

WALNUT NUTTER BUTTER FAT BOMBS

Prep Time: 15 minutes
Cooking Time: 1 hour & 15 minutes
Servings: 8

Nutritional Info (Estimated Amount Per Serving)

- 300 Calories

- 272 Calories from Fat

- 30g Total Fat

- 16g Saturated Fat

- 0g Trans Fat

- 3.5g Polyunsaturated Fat

- 8.1g Monounsaturated Fat

- 16mg Cholesterol

- 76mg Sodium

- 147mg Potassium

- 7.1g Total Carbohydrates

- 2g Dietary Fiber

- 2.4g Sugars

- 3.8g Protein

INGREDIENTS

- ½ cup almond butter

- 4 tbsp. unsalted butter

- 2 tbsp. chopped walnuts

- ½ cup coconut oil

- Melted dark chocolate to taste

- 6 drops of liquid stevia or to taste

- Sea salt to taste

DIRECTIONS

1. Combine the entire ingredients in a small bowl or dish & heat for 30 seconds in the microwave, until warm. Whisk until blended well.

2. Pour the mixture into molds, cupcake liners or muffin tins & place them into a freezer; let chill for an hour, until firm.

3. Once set; carefully remove the fat bombs from molds and top each first with the melted dark or sugar free chocolate & then walnut pieces.

ALMOND JOY
FAT BOMBS

Prep Time: 15 minutes
Cooking Time: 2 hours & 20 minutes
Servings: 15

Nutritional Info (Estimated Amount Per Serving)

- 30 Calories

- 22 Calories from Fat

- 2.4g Total Fat

- 1.4g Saturated Fat

- 0g Trans Fat

- 0.2g Polyunsaturated Fat

- 0.6g Monounsaturated Fat

- 0.3mg Cholesterol

- 12mg Sodium

- 20mg Potassium

- 2g Total Carbohydrates

- 0.3g Dietary Fiber

- 1.3g Sugars

- 0.4g Protein

INGREDIENTS

- 15 almonds

- 1 tbsp. coconut oil

- ¼ cup coconut, shredded

- 1 tbsp. erythritol

- ½ chocolate bar recipe, low-carb

DIRECTIONS

1. Prepare the Chocolate Bar recipe in advance, but ensure that you don't add it into the mold.

2. Pour approximately ½ tsp. of the chocolate mixture into each candy molds & then add an almond to every mold. Place the molds into a freezer and let chill for a couple of minutes.

3. Now, mix the coconut oil together with shredded coconut; mix well and then add in the erythritol; give everything a good stir until evenly mixed.

4. Add a tsp. of the coconut mixture to candy molds; gently press and make a flat top layer.

5. Let chill in the freezer until solidifies, for 5 to 7 minutes.

6. Top the candies molds with the leftover chocolate mixture; smoothing the top out. Freeze for an hour, until set.

7. Once done; carefully remove the fat-bombs from the molds. Serve immediately and enjoy.

CARAMEL APPLE PIE FAT BOMB

Prep Time: 10 minutes
Cooking Time: 40 minutes
Servings: 8

Nutritional Info (Estimated Amount Per Serving)

- 169 Calories

- 127 Calories from Fat

- 14g Total Fat

- 12g Saturated Fat

- 0g Trans Fat

- 0.2g Polyunsaturated Fat

- 0.7g Monounsaturated Fat

- 0mg Cholesterol

- 24mg Sodium

- 139mg Potassium

- 17g Total Carbohydrates

- 3.9g Dietary Fiber

- 7.1g Sugars

- 1.3g Protein

INGREDIENTS

- 2 green apples, organic, medium, cored & sliced

- 1 can coconut cream (5.4oz)

- 20 drops of liquid stevia, preferably English toffee

- ½ cup coconut butter

- 1 tsp. cinnamon

- 2 tbsp. coconut oil

- A pinch of sea salt

DIRECTIONS

1. Over moderate heat settings in a large skillet heat the coconut oils until melted and then sauté the apples until soft, for a couple of minutes. Add in the cinnamon; give everything a good stir until the sautéed apples are evenly coated.

2. Now, combine the remaining ingredients together in a blender; blend until liquefied, on high settings. Pour the mixture into the silicon molds.

3. Place the filled molds into the freezer and let chill until firm, for an hour.

4. Once done; carefully remove the fat-bombs from the molds. Serve immediately and enjoy.

COCONUT BERRY
FAT BOMBS

Prep Time: 15 minutes
Cooking Time: 55 minutes
Servings: 12

Nutritional Info (Estimated Amount Per Serving)

- 171 Calories

- 162 Calories from Fat

- 18g Total Fat

- 15g Saturated Fat

- 0g Trans Fat

- 0.3g Polyunsaturated Fat

- 1.2g Monounsaturated Fat

- 0mg Cholesterol

- 0.2mg Sodium

- 9.4mg Potassium

- 2.1g Total Carbohydrates

- 0.2g Dietary Fiber

- 1.8g Sugars

- 0.1g Protein

INGREDIENTS

- ½ cup mixed berries, frozen such as blueberries, raspberries, strawberries, pomegranates and cherries

- 1 cup coconut oil, refined

- 14 drops of liquid stevia or honey

- 1 tsp. vanilla extract

DIRECTIONS

1. Over moderate heat settings in a large saucepan; heat the coconut oil until melted. In the meantime; process the frozen fruit briefly in a food processor until chopped into very small pieces.

2. Add stevia and vanilla extract to the food processor.

3. Add melted coconut oil into the food processor with the fruit & remaining ingredients; process on high settings until evenly mixed. Continue to mix until the entire fruit is blended smoothly into oil.

4. Scoop the prepared mixture into molds.

5. Place the molds into the freezer and let chill for 30 minutes, until firm up. Once done; carefully remove the fat-bombs from molds. Serve immediately and enjoy.

MOCHA ICE BOMBS

Prep Time: 15 minutes
Cooking Time: 2 hours & 20 minutes
Servings: 12

Nutritional Info (Estimated Amount Per Serving)

- 147 Calories

- 122 Calories from Fat

- 14g Total Fat

- 8g Saturated Fat

- 0.2g Trans Fat

- 0.5g Polyunsaturated Fat

- 3.6g Monounsaturated Fat

- 29mg Cholesterol

- 92mg Sodium

- 48mg Potassium

- 5.4g Total Carbohydrates

- 0.4g Dietary Fiber

- 4.2g Sugars

- 1.6g Protein

INGREDIENTS

For Mocha Ice Bombs:

- 60 ml strong coffee chilled

- 2 tbsp. cocoa unsweetened

- 240 g mascarpone or cream cheese

- 4 tbsp. sweetener, powdered

For Chocolate Coating:

- 28 g melted cocoa butter

- 70 g melted chocolate, preferably 90%

DIRECTIONS

1. Add coffee together with the mascarpone or cream cheese, unsweetened cocoa & sweetener in a food processor; process on high settings until smooth, for a minute or two.

2. Roll approximately 2 tbsp. of the mocha ice bomb mixture and form 12 ice bombs; arrange them onto a clean plate or tray lined with the baking parchment.

For Chocolate Coating

1. Thoroughly combine the cocoa butter with melted chocolate; mix well.

2. Roll every prepared ice bomb into the chocolate coating; arrange them on the lined plate/tray again.

3. Place in a freezer and let chill until set, for a couple of hours

COOKIE DOUGH FAT BOMBS

Prep Time: 5 minutes
Cooking Time: 1 hour & 15 minutes
Servings: 10

Nutritional Info (Estimated Amount Per Serving)

- 215 Calories

- 182 Calories from Fat

- 20g Total Fat

- 11g Saturated Fat

- 0g Trans Fat

- 2.1g Polyunsaturated Fat

- 5.9g Monounsaturated Fat

- 0.5mg Cholesterol

- 1.9mg Sodium

- 140mg Potassium

- 7.1g Total Carbohydrates

- 2.1g Dietary Fiber

- 3.4g Sugars

- 3.4g Protein

INGREDIENTS

- ¼ cup finely chopped dark chocolate, preferably honey-sweetened

- ¾ cup almond flour

- 1 tbsp. liquid stevia

- ¼ cup Almond butter, organic

- ½ cup melted coconut oil, organic

DIRECTIONS

1. Combine coconut oil together with almond flour, almond butter, and maple syrup in a large bowl; mix well.

2. Slowly fold in the chocolate; mix well.

3. Pour the mixture into a loaf pan & freeze for an hour, until just set.

4. Just before serving; cut into squares. Serve and enjoy.

CHOCOLATES WITH MACADAMIA & SEA SALT FAT BOMBS

Prep Time: 15 minutes
Cooking Time: 15 minutes
Servings: 12

Nutritional Info (Estimated Amount Per Serving)

- 125 Calories

- 117 Calories from Fat

- 13g Total Fat

- 9.6g Saturated Fat

- 0g Trans Fat

- 0.2g Polyunsaturated Fat

- 2g Monounsaturated Fat

- 0mg Cholesterol

- 49mg Sodium

- 7.7mg Potassium

- 1.7g Total Carbohydrates

- 0.6g Dietary Fiber

- 0.1g Sugars

- 0.6g Protein

INGREDIENTS

- 3 tbsp. coarsely chopped macadamia nuts

- 5 tbsp. cocoa powder, unsweetened

- 10 tbsp. coconut oil

- Coarse Sea Salt to taste

- 2 g granulated stevia

DIRECTIONS

1. Over moderate heat settings in a large saucepan; heat the coconut oil until melted.

2. Add granulated Stevia and cocoa powder; give everything a good stir and then remove the pan from heat.

3. Now, evenly spoon the prepared mixture into the silicone candy molds.

4. Refrigerate until the mixture resembles a gel-like consistency and thickens.

5. Sprinkle each well with the macadamia nuts; pressing the nuts down. Place the mold into the refrigerator again and let chill until hardened completely.

6. Once done, remove the chocolates from molds and place on a cupcake liner or dish, preferably right side up.

7. Let sit until the surface starts to glisten, at room temperature. Sprinkle a pinch of course sea salt over each chocolate fat-bomb. Serve immediately and enjoy.

DAIRY-FREE CINNAMON ROLL CHEESECAKE FAT BOMBS

Prep Time: 10 minutes
Cooking Time: 20 minutes
Servings: 12

Nutritional Info (Estimated Amount Per Serving)

- 159 Calories
- 138 Calories from Fat
- 15g Total Fat
- 9.2g Saturated Fat
- 0g Trans Fat
- 1g Polyunsaturated Fat
- 3.7g Monounsaturated Fat
- 22mg Cholesterol
- 75mg Sodium
- 67mg Potassium
- 4g Total Carbohydrates
- 1.1g Dietary Fiber
- 1.1g Sugars
- 2.4g Protein

INGREDIENTS

For Almond Flour Center:

- 1 tbsp. Erythritol

- 2 tbsp. Non-dairy coconut oil

- ½ cup Almond flour, raw

For Cream Cheese Layer:

- 8 oz. cream cheese, dairy-free

- 2 tsp. ground cinnamon

- 6 tbsp. Erythritol

- 3 tbsp. Non-dairy coconut oil

For Sugar-Cinnamon Topping:

- 2 tsp. ground cinnamon

- ¼ cup erythritol

DIRECTIONS

1. In a small bowl; combine almond flour together with erythritol, and coconut oil; Knead until well incorporated using clean hands. Evenly separate the prepared mixture into 12 pieces; roll each piece into ball. Arrange the balls on a cookie sheet lined with a parchment paper & place the sheet in a freezer until ready to use.

2. In the meantime, in a small bowl; combine cream cheese together with erythritol and coconut oil. Divide the mixture evenly between 2 bowls. Add ground cinnamon in one of the cream cheese bowls; mix until well incorporated and then place in the freezer; let chill for an hour.

3. Now, combining the sugar-cinnamon topping ingredients

together in a small bowl; mix well & set aside until ready to use.

4. Now, scoop a tsp. of plain cream cheese mixture & a tsp. of cream cheese-cinnamon mixture onto a parchment piece. Place the prepared almond flour balls in the middle. Roll until evenly coated. Now, place in the coated balls in the bowl with sugar-cinnamon mixture & roll until coated as well.

5. Arrange the ball over the parchment paper again & place in the freezer.

6. Let chill for 20 minutes. Serve immediately and enjoy.

JALAPENO POPPERS FAT BOMBS

Prep Time: 15 minutes
Cooking Time: 30 minutes
Servings: 6

Nutritional Info (Estimated Amount Per Serving)

- 233 Calories

- 209 Calories from Fat

- 23g Total Fat

- 12g Saturated Fat

- 0g Trans Fat

- 1.9g Polyunsaturated Fat

- 7.7g Monounsaturated Fat

- 56mg Cholesterol

- 212mg Sodium

- 75mg Potassium

- 1.5g Total Carbohydrates

- 0.1g Dietary Fiber

- 1g Sugars

- 4.9g Protein

INGREDIENTS

- 2 jalapeño peppers, halved, seeded & chopped finely

- ¼ cup ghee or unsalted butter, at room temperature

- 3.5 ounces cream cheese, full-fat, at room temperature

- ¼ cup Cheddar cheese or Gruyère cheese, grated

- 4 bacon slices (4.2 oz)

DIRECTIONS

1. Line a rimmed baking sheet (preferably large-sized) with the parchment paper and preheat your oven to 325 F in advance.

2. Mash cream cheese together with ghee or butter in a large bowl; mash well until completely smooth (Feel free to use food processor for this step).

3. Arrange the bacon slices over the parchment paper baking sheet; make sure you don't over-crowd them.

4. Now, place the sheet with the bacon slices in the oven & cook until crispy, for approximately half an hour.

5. Once done; remove the baking sheet from oven; set aside at room temperature to cool, until easy to handle. Crumble the cooked bacon slices in a bowl; set aside until ready to use.

6. Add the Cheddar cheese or Gruyère together with bacon grease, and jalapeños to the butter-cream cheese mixture. Mix until combined well. Place the bowl into a refrigerator and let chill until set, for approximately an hour.

7. Form six fat bombs from the mixture & arrange them on a clean plate lined with parchment paper. Roll the prepared fat-bombs in the crumbled bacon (one by one) until coated well. Serve immediately and enjoy.

SAVORY PIZZA
FAT BOMBS

Prep Time: 35 minutes
Cooking Time: 2 hours
Servings: 6

Nutritional Info (Estimated Amount Per Serving)

- 118 Calories

- 100 Calories from Fat

- 11g Total Fat

- 5.1g Saturated Fat

- 0.1g Trans Fat

- 0.7g Polyunsaturated Fat

- 4.3g Monounsaturated Fat

- 24mg Cholesterol

- 195mg Sodium

- 103mg Potassium

- 2.5g Total Carbohydrates

- 0.4g Dietary Fiber

- 1.4g Sugars

- 2.6g Protein

INGREDIENTS

- 4 oz. cream cheese

- 2 tbsp. tomato pesto, preferably sun-dried

- 8 black olives, pitted, diced into small pieces

- 2 tbsp. basil, fresh & chopped

- Pepper and salt to taste

- 14 pepperoni slices, diced into small pieces

DIRECTIONS

1. Mix tomato pesto together with cream cheese, and basil in a large bowl; mix well.

2. Now, add diced pepperoni and olives into the tomato pesto-cream cheese mixture; mix again until combined well.

3. Form six even-sized balls from the mixture and garnish each bowl with basil, pepperoni, and olive. Serve immediately and enjoy.

SAVORY SALMON
FAT BOMBS

Prep Time: 10 minutes
Cooking Time: 1 hour & 15 minutes
Servings: 6

Nutritional Info (Estimated Amount Per Serving)

- 177 Calories

- 163 Calories from Fat

- 18g Total Fat

- 11g Saturated Fat

- 0.4g Trans Fat

- 1g Polyunsaturated Fat

- 4.9g Monounsaturated Fat

- 53mg Cholesterol

- 166mg Sodium

- 61mg Potassium

- 1.2g Total Carbohydrates

- 0g Dietary Fiber

- 0.8g Sugars

- 3g Protein

INGREDIENTS

- ½ package smoked mackerel or smoked salmon

- 1-2 tbsp. dill, freshly chopped or 1 tsp dried

- 1/3 cup grass-fed butter

- 1 tbsp. lemon juice, fresh

- ½ cup cream cheese, full-fat

- A pinch of Himalayan pink salt

DIRECTIONS

1. Place smoked salmon together with butter, and cream cheese in a food processor. Now, add dill and freshly squeezed lemon juice in the food processor; pulse on high settings until completely smooth.

2. Line a large-sized tray with the parchment paper & form six fat-bombs from the mixture. Garnish each fat-bomb with some more dill & then place the tray in a fridge; let chill until firm, for an hour.

CHEESE, BACON CAULIFLOWER FAT BOMBS

Prep Time: 5 minutes
Cooking Time: 15 minute
Servings: 10

Nutritional Info (Estimated Amount Per Serving)

- 535 Calories

- 360 Calories from Fat

- 40g Total Fat

- 19g Saturated Fat

- 0.4g Trans Fat

- 4.1g Polyunsaturated Fat

- 14g Monounsaturated Fat

- 110mg Cholesterol

- 1495mg Sodium

- 491mg Potassium

- 12g Total Carbohydrates

- 1.4g Dietary Fiber

- 2.3g Sugars

- 31g Protein

INGREDIENTS

- 5 cups riced cauliflower
- 1 lb. bacon, cooked & crumbled
- 8 oz cream cheese, softened
- 4 oz. goat cheese
- 1 ½ cup grated parmesan cheese, divided
- ½ cup sharp cheddar cheese
- ½ cup sharp garlic white cheddar cheese
- 1 cup crushed pork rinds
- ½ cup panko
- 3 cloves garlic, minced
- 1 tsp. Italian seasoning, divided
- 1 tsp. onion powder
- 1 tsp. garlic powder
- ½ tsp. sea salt
- ½ tsp. black pepper
- Oil

DIRECTIONS

1. Combine bacon together with minced garlic, riced cauliflower, goat cheese, ½ cup grated Parmesan, softened cream cheese, garlic white cheddar cheese, sharp cheddar cheese, ½ tsp. Italian seasoning, pepper and sea salt in a large-sized mixing bowl. Mix until incorporated well.

2. Place the bowl in a refrigerator and let chill until firm, for a couple of hours.

3. Now, for breading: Mix the crushed pork rinds together with Panko, leftover 1 cup Parmesan cheese, Italian seasoning, garlic powder, and onion powder.

4. Once the cauliflower mixture is firm, form approximately 30 even-sized balls from the mixture by rolling it between your palms. Freeze for a minimum period of 3 hours or for overnight.

5. Fill a large pan with 1" of oil and heat it over medium to high settings until hot but not smoky.

6. Roll each formed ball into the breading mixture using your hands, until coated well. Work in batches and drop the coated balls into the hot oil. Fry until all sides turn golden brown, flipping as required.

7. Remove the cooked balls from oil; place them on paper towel and let cool. Served these with ranch dressing and low-carb marinara.

EGG & BACON
FAT BOMBS

Prep Time: 10 minutes
Cooking Time: 45 minutes
Servings: 6

Nutritional Info (Estimated Amount Per Serving)

- 209 Calories

- 189 Calories from Fat

- 21g Total Fat

- 8.8g Saturated Fat

- 0g Trans Fat

- 3.9g Polyunsaturated Fat

- 7.1g Monounsaturated Fat

- 98mg Cholesterol

- 241mg Sodium

- 66mg Potassium

- 0.6g Total Carbohydrates

- 0.1g Dietary Fiber

- 0.3g Sugars

- 4.6g Protein

INGREDIENTS

- 4 bacon slices, large (4.2 oz)

- 2 tbsp. mayonnaise

- ¼ cup ghee or butter, softened at room temperature; cut into small pieces

- 2 eggs, large, organic or free-range

- ¼ tsp. Himalayan pink salt or to taste

- Freshly ground black pepper

DIRECTIONS

1. Line a large-sized baking tray with the baking paper & preheat your oven to 375 F in advance. Arrange the bacon strips over the baking paper; don't over-crowd them. Now, cook in the preheated oven until turns golden brown, for 10 to 15 minutes. When done, immediately remove the baking tray from the oven; set aside at room temperature to cool.

2. In the meantime; fill a small-sized saucepan with water (enough to cover the eggs). Sprinkle a pinch of salt and add the eggs and bring to a boil, over moderate heat settings. Continue to boil the eggs for 8 to 10 minutes. When done, remove the boiled eggs from heat & place them in a bowl with cold water until easy to handle. When done, peel the shells off.

3. Add peeled & quartered eggs with butter in a large bowl; mash well with a large fork.

4. Add mayonnaise and then season with pepper and salt to taste; mix well. Add bacon grease & continue to mix. Place the bowl in a fridge and let chill until solid & you can easily form the fat bombs from the mixture, for half an hour.

5. Add the cooked bacon in a large bowl and crumble into small pieces. Remove the egg mixture from fridge and form six even-sized balls. Roll each formed ball into the crumbled bacon & arrange them on a tray. Let chill in the fridge again.

BACON & GUACAMOLE FAT BOMBS

Prep Time: 10 minutes
Cooking Time: 40 minutes
Servings: 6

Nutritional Info (Estimated Amount Per Serving)

- 360 Calories

- 319 Calories from Fat

- 35g Total Fat

- 16g Saturated Fat

- 0.1g Trans Fat

- 3.5g Polyunsaturated Fat

- 14g Monounsaturated Fat

- 68mg Cholesterol

- 381mg Sodium

- 283mg Potassium

- 6.5g Total Carbohydrates

- 2.2g Dietary Fiber

- 1.8g Sugars

- 5.9g Protein

INGREDIENTS

- 4 bacon slices, large
- ½ avocado, large; halved, deseeded & peeled
- 1 tbsp. lime juice, freshly squeezed
- 2 garlic cloves, crushed
- 1 chili pepper, small, chopped finely
- ½ white onion, small, diced
- 1-2 tbsp. cilantro, freshly chopped
- ¼ cup ghee or butter, softened at room temperature
- Freshly ground cayenne or black pepper
- ¼ tsp. Himalayan pink salt or to taste

DIRECTIONS

1. Line a large-sized baking tray with the baking paper and then preheat your oven to 375 F in advance. Arrange the bacon strips over the baking paper; don't over-crowd the pieces. Cook in the preheated oven until turn golden brown, for 10 to 15 minutes. When the slices are cooked to your likings, remove the baking tray immediately from oven; set aside at room temperature to cool down.

2. Place the halved avocado together with chili pepper, butter, crushed garlic, lime juice, and cilantro into a large bowl & then season with pepper and salt to taste.

3. Using a large fork or potato masher; mash until combined well. Add in the diced onion; mix again.

4. Add the bacon grease; mix well. Using a foil; cover the bowl & place in a fridge; let chill for several minutes.

5. For breading: crumble the bacon into pieces, preferably small-sized. Remove the bowl with guacamole mixture from fridge; form six even sized balls using your palms. Roll each formed ball into the crumbled bacon & arrange them on a tray. Let chill in the fridge again until ready to serve.

BAKED BRIE & PECAN PROSCIUTTO SAVORY FAT BOMBS

Prep Time: 15 minute
Cooking Time: 15 minute
Servings: 4

Nutritional Info (Estimated Amount Per Serving)

- 46 Calories

- 35 Calories from Fat

- 3.9g Total Fat

- 1.5g Saturated Fat

- 0g Trans Fat

- 0.6g Polyunsaturated Fat

- 1.6g Monounsaturated Fat

- 9.6mg Cholesterol

- 140mg Sodium

- 39mg Potassium

- 0.4g Total Carbohydrates

- 0.2g Dietary Fiber

- 0.1g Sugars

- 2.7g Protein

INGREDIENTS

- 6 pecan halves, approximately ⅓ ounce

- 1 slice of prosciutto, approximately ½ ounce; sliced & fold it in half

- ⅛ tsp. black pepper

- 1 ounce Brie cheese, full-fat; chopped in small cubes, don't remove the white skin

DIRECTIONS

1. Preheat your oven to 350 F in advance. Place the sliced prosciutto in the hole of a muffin tin (approximately 1 ½" deep & 2 ½" wide).

2. Place the chopped Brie in the cup with prosciutto.

3. Now, add the pecan halves.

4. Bake in the preheated oven until prosciutto is cooked and Brie is melted, for 10 to 12 minutes.

5. Before removing; let cool for several minutes at room temperature.

WHITE CHOCOLATE BUTTER PECAN FAT BOMBS

Prep Time: 10 minutes
Cooking Time: 40 minutes
Servings: 5

Nutritional Info (Estimated Amount Per Serving)

- 223 Calories

- 184 Calories from Fat

- 20g Total Fat

- 12g Saturated Fat

- 0g Trans Fat

- 1g Polyunsaturated Fat

- 5.8g Monounsaturated Fat

- 54mg Cholesterol

- 265mg Sodium

- 331mg Potassium

- 7.7g Total Carbohydrates

- 1.9g Dietary Fiber

- 3.6g Sugars

- 4.3g Protein

INGREDIENTS

- 5 tbsp. grated parmesan cheese (0.9 oz)

- 4 pieces tomatoes, sun-dried, drained (0.4 oz)

- ½ cup full-fat cream cheese (3.5 oz)

- 2-3 tbsp. herbs, freshly chopped (such as thyme, oregano and basil)

- ¼ cup ghee or butter, softened at room temperature; cut butter into thin-sized pieces

- 4 kalamata olives, pitted (0.4 oz)

- Freshly ground black pepper

- 2 garlic cloves, crushed

- ¼ tsp. pink Himalayan salt or to taste

DIRECTIONS

1. Add the butter cubes and cream cheese in a bowl. Leave it on a kitchen counter until soften, for half an hour. Mash well using a large fork until combined well. Add in the kalamata olives and sun-dried tomatoes.

2. Add in the herbs followed by the crushed garlic; mix well and then season with pepper and salt. Mix well & then place in a fridge until solidify, for half an hour.

3. After half an hour; remove the cheese mixture & form 5 even-sized balls. Now, roll each ball into the grated parmesan cheese; arranging them on a clean plate.

4. Serve immediately and enjoy.

BACON HERB CREAM CHEESE DIP AKA SAVORY FAT BOMB

Prep Time: 15 minutes
Cooking Time: 45 minutes
Servings: 6

Nutritional Info (Estimated Amount Per Serving)

- 254 Calories

- 206 Calories from Fat

- 23g Total Fat

- 9.5g Saturated Fat

- 0.1g Trans Fat

- 2.8g Polyunsaturated Fat

- 9.2g Monounsaturated Fat

- 31mg Cholesterol

- 301mg Sodium

- 124mg Potassium

- 5.9g Total Carbohydrates

- 0.6g Dietary Fiber

- 2.9g Sugars

- 6.2g Protein

INGREDIENTS

- ¼ cup bacon bits

- 1 cup yogurt cream cheese or kefir cream cheese, at room temperature

- ½ cup bacon fat, at room temperature

- 2 garlic cloves

- 1 tsp. oregano, fresh, chopped

- ½ cup grated Parmesan cheese

- Freshly cracked pepper and salt, to taste

DIRECTIONS

1. Process the cream cheese in a food processor until loosen up. Add in the garlic cloves and then sprinkle a small amount of pepper and salt. Process again.

2. Gradually, pour a small stream of liquid bacon fat and process until completely incorporated.

3. Place the mixture into a large bowl.

4. Add the leftover ingredients into the mixture and then fold. Evenly divide the mixture into six portions & refrigerate. Serve and enjoy.

DELICIOUS PECANS FAT BOMBS

Prep Time: 2 minutes
Cooking Time: 2 minutes
Servings: 2

Nutritional Info (Estimated Amount Per Serving)

- 46 Calories

- 45 Calories from Fat

- 5g Total Fat

- 2g Saturated Fat

- 0g Trans Fat

- 0.8g Polyunsaturated Fat

- 2g Monounsaturated Fat

- 7.6mg Cholesterol

- 66mg Sodium

- 13mg Potassium

- 0.4g Total Carbohydrates

- 0.3g Dietary Fiber

- 0.1g Sugars

- 0.3g Protein

INGREDIENTS

- 4 toasted pecan halves

- ½ tbsp. unsalted butter, grass-fed

- A pinch of best quality sea salt

DIRECTIONS

1. Spread ½ of the unsalted butter between 2 halves of pecan. Sprinkle a very small quantity of sea salt over the top. Serve and enjoy.

SAVORY SESAME FAT BOMBS

Prep Time: 10 minutes
Cooking Time: 30 minutes
Servings: 4

Nutritional Info (Estimated Amount Per Serving)

- 271 Calories

- 274 Calories from Fat

- 30g Total Fat

- 15g Saturated Fat

- 0g Trans Fat

- 4g Polyunsaturated Fat

- 9.6g Monounsaturated Fat

- 61mg Cholesterol

- 586mg Sodium

- 14mg Potassium

- 0.4g Total Carbohydrates

- 0.2g Dietary Fiber

- 0g Sugars

- 0.5g Protein

INGREDIENTS

- 2 tsp. sesame seeds, toasted

- 1 tsp. sea salt

- 2 tbsp. sesame oil

- ¼ tsp. chili flakes

- 4 oz. unsalted butter, at room temperature

DIRECTIONS

1. Roast the sesame seeds over moderate heat settings in a dry, hot pan until golden brown & begin popping, for a few minutes, stirring frequently; don't let them burn. Transfer the roasted seeds immediately to a shallow bowl or large plate; set aside.

2. Now, mix sesame oil together with butter, salt and chili flakes in a bowl, preferably small-sized. Place the bowl in a fridge for several minutes.

3. Form walnut sized balls from the butter mixture. Roll each ball in the toasted sesame seeds. Serve immediately and enjoy or store them in an air-tight container in the freezer or fridge.

JALAPENO POPPER FAT BOMB

Prep Time: 10 minutes
Cooking Time: 25 minutes
Servings: 3

Nutritional Info (Estimated Amount Per Serving)

- 219 Calories

- 188 Calories from Fat

- 21g Total Fat

- 9.5g Saturated Fat

- 0g Trans Fat

- 2.2g Polyunsaturated Fat

- 7.4g Monounsaturated Fat

- 47mg Cholesterol

- 275mg Sodium

- 111mg Potassium

- 2.6g Total Carbohydrates

- 0.2g Dietary Fiber

- 1.6g Sugars

- 5.4g Protein

INGREDIENTS

- 3 bacon slices

- ¼ tsp. garlic powder

- 1 jalapeno pepper, medium; de-seeded & dice into thin pieces

- ½ tsp. parsley, dried

- 3 ounces cream cheese

- ¼ tsp. onion powder

- Pepper & salt to taste

DIRECTIONS

1. Fry three bacon slices until crisp, over moderate heat settings in a large pan.

2. Remove the crisped bacon from pan; keeping the grease in the pan. Set aside at room temperature and let cool.

3. Combine jalapeno together with cream cheese & spices in a large bowl. Season with pepper and salt to taste.

4. Add in the bacon fat; mix well until you get solid mixture like consistency.

5. Crumble the bacon & set on a clean plate. Using your hand; roll the cream cheese mixture into balls and then roll each ball into the crumbled bacon.

SAVORY KETO JALAPENO, CHEESE & BACON BITE FAT BOMBS

Prep Time: 10 minutes
Cooking Time: 3 hours & 30 minutes
Servings: 18

Nutritional Info (Estimated Amount Per Serving)

- 167 Calories
- 151 Calories from Fat
- 17g Total Fat
- 9.7g Saturated Fat
- 0.1g Trans Fat
- 1.1g Polyunsaturated Fat
- 4.5g Monounsaturated Fat
- 26mg Cholesterol
- 127mg Sodium
- 41mg Potassium
- 1.2g Total Carbohydrates
- 0.1g Dietary Fiber
- 0.7g Sugars
- 3g Protein

INGREDIENTS

- 4 bacon slices, chopped & cooked, reserve the grease
- 8 ounces cream cheese, full-fat or dripped yogurt cheese (1 cup)
- 2 ounces bacon grease (1/3 cup)
- 4 ounces cheddar cheese, shredded (½ cup loosely filled)
- 3 ounces expeller-pressed coconut oil, melted (1/3 cup plus 1 tbsp.)
- 4 jalapeno peppers, seeds & stems removed; rinsed & finely diced

DIRECTIONS

1. Cook the bacon slices in a medium skillet, over medium heat settings.

2. Combine cheddar cheese together with cream cheese, melted coconut oil, diced Jalapeno, and bacon grease. Don't add the cooked bacon.

3. Press the cream cheese mixture into a loaf pan lined with parchment & let chill until firm, for a couple of hours.

4. For serving: set the bacon pieces aside.

5. Remove the cream cheese mixture from loaf pan & cut into 18 even-sized pieces.

6. Gently roll the pieces into balls & then roll each ball into the crumbled bacon.

7. Enjoy immediately & enjoy.

WALDORF SALAD FAT BOMBS

Prep Time: 15 minutes
Cooking Time: 40 minutes
Servings: 8

Nutritional Info (Estimated Amount Per Serving)

- 161 Calories

- 140 Calories from Fat

- 16g Total Fat

- 6.2g Saturated Fat

- 0g Trans Fat

- 2.2g Polyunsaturated Fat

- 6.1g Monounsaturated Fat

- 25mg Cholesterol

- 131mg Sodium

- 88mg Potassium

- 3.5g Total Carbohydrates

- 1.1g Dietary Fiber

- 1.8g Sugars

- 3.3g Protein

INGREDIENTS

- ½ green apple, small, diced into ½" pieces

- 3 ounces cream cheese, full-fat, at room temperature (85 g)

- 2/3 cup walnuts or pecans, chopped roughly

- 2 tbsp. ghee or unsalted butter, at room temperature

- ¼ tsp. onion powder

- 2 tbsp. spring onion or chives, fresh chopped

- ½ cup blue cheese, crumbled

- Pepper & salt, to taste

- ¼ tsp. garlic powder

DIRECTIONS

1. Process cream cheese together with ghee or butter in a food processor or mash in a large bowl until completely smooth.

2. Add in the apple, crumbled blue cheese, onion powder, garlic powder & chives. Give everything a good stir until evenly combined and then season with pepper and salt to taste. Refrigerate until set, for 20 to 30 minutes.

3. Divide the mixture evenly into six balls using an ice cream scoop or a large spoon. Roll each ball into the bowl with walnuts or pecans. Serve immediately and enjoy.

CHEESY BACON BOMBS

Prep Time: 10 minutes
Cooking Time: 55 minutes
Servings: 20

Nutritional Info (Estimated Amount Per Serving)

- 229 Calories

- 204 Calories from Fat

- 23g Total Fat

- 5.7g Saturated Fat

- 0.2g Trans Fat

- 3.3g Polyunsaturated Fat

- 12g Monounsaturated Fat

- 34mg Cholesterol

- 215mg Sodium

- 80mg Potassium

- 2.3g Total Carbohydrates

- 1.2g Dietary Fiber

- 0.3g Sugars

- 5.3g Protein

INGREDIENTS

- 10 bacon slices

- 8 ounces mozzarella cheese

- ¼ tsp. black pepper

- 3 tbsp. Psyllium Husk Powder

- 1/8 tsp. onion powder

- 1 egg, large

- 4 tbsp. almond flour

- 1/8 tsp. garlic powder

- 4 tbsp. butter, melted

- 1 cup lard, oil or tallow for frying

- ¼ tsp. salt

DIRECTIONS

1. Microwave the cheese until gooey and melted, for 45 to 60 seconds.

2. Heat 1 tbsp. of butter in a microwave until it's completely melted, for 15-20 seconds. Add half of the Mozzarella cheese to a large bowl. Add butter and egg to the mixture; mix well.

3. Add 3 tbsp. of psyllium husk, 4 tbsp. of almond flour & the remaining spices to the mixture. Mix well & place it onto a silpat. Form rectangle from the dough; using your hands or rolling the dough.

4. Spread the remaining cheese over half of the dough & fold lengthwise. Now, form a square shape by again folding the dough vertically.

5. Using your fingers; crimp the edges & press the dough together into a rectangle. Cut the dough into 20 even-sized squares using a sharp knife.

6. Cut each bacon slice in half and then lay the square at the end. Tightly roll the dough into the bacon until the ends are just overlapping.

7. Secure the bacon using a toothpick. Now, over moderately high heat settings; heat up the lard, oil, or tallow and slowly fry the cheesy bacon bombs.

8. Place the fired fat-bombs over a paper towel; drain & let cool at room temperature. Serve immediately and enjoy.

AVOCADO TUNA MELT BITES

Prep Time: 25 minutes
Cooking Time: 25 minutes
Servings: 12

Nutritional Info (Estimated Amount Per Serving)

- 189 Calories

- 153 Calories from Fat

- 17g Total Fat

- 8.9g Saturated Fat

- 0g Trans Fat

- 3.1g Polyunsaturated Fat

- 3.8g Monounsaturated Fat

- 14mg Cholesterol

- 157mg Sodium

- 143mg Potassium

- 2.1g Total Carbohydrates

- 1.2g Dietary Fiber

- 0.2g Sugars

- 7.1g Protein

INGREDIENTS

- ¼ cup mayonnaise

- 10 ounces tuna, canned, drained

- ½ tsp. garlic powder

- ¼ tsp. onion powder

- 1 avocado, medium, sliced in half, pit removed, cubed

- 1/3 cup almond flour

- ¼ cup Parmesan cheese

- ½ cup coconut oil

- Pepper and salt to taste

DIRECTIONS

1. Add tuna to a container, preferably large-sized.

2. Now, add parmesan cheese together with mayonnaise & spices to the container with tuna; mix well.

3. Add avocado; fold everything together; don't mash the avocado.

4. Form approximately 12 even-sized balls from the tuna mixture & then roll each prepared ball into the almond flour; ensure that the flour covers the balls completely; set aside at room temperature.

5. Now, over moderate heat settings in a large pan; heat the coconut oil. Once hot, work in batches and slowly add the prepared tuna balls; fry for a couple of minutes on all sides, until crisp.

6. Remove; serve immediately and enjoy.

KETO
TUNA MELTS

Prep Time: 15 minutes
Cooking Time: 25 minutes
Servings: 6

Nutritional Info (Estimated Amount Per Serving)

- 250 Calories

- 184 Calories from Fat

- 20g Total Fat

- 8.1g Saturated Fat

- 0.4g Trans Fat

- 5.2g Polyunsaturated Fat

- 5.4g Monounsaturated Fat

- 109mg Cholesterol

- 649mg Sodium

- 115mg Potassium

- 1.5g Total Carbohydrates

- 0g Dietary Fiber

- 0.6g Sugars

- 14g Protein

INGREDIENTS

- 5 oz. can of tuna fish; drained

- 2 eggs, large

- ¼ cup mayo

- 1 ½ cups shredded cheese

- ¼ cup sour cream

- 1 tsp. parsley, fresh, chopped

- ¾ tsp. table salt or sea salt to taste

DIRECTIONS

1. Add the canned tuna fish together with sour cream, mayo, cheese, eggs, parsley, pepper and salt in a medium-sized bowl; mix well.

2. Evenly divide the tuna mixture in a cupcake tin, preferably lightly-greased.

3. Bake for 20 to 25 minutes at 350 F.

4. Once done; set aside and let cool. Serve and enjoy.

SALMON PATE
FAT BOMBS

Prep Time: 15 minutes
Cooking Time: 15 minutes
Servings: 6

Nutritional Info (Estimated Amount Per Serving)

- 332 Calories

- 296 Calories from Fat

- 33g Total Fat

- 20g Saturated Fat

- 0g Trans Fat

- 1.5g Polyunsaturated Fat

- 9.4g Monounsaturated Fat

- 94mg Cholesterol

- 675mg Sodium

- 132mg Potassium

- 2.8g Total Carbohydrates

- 0.4g Dietary Fiber

- 1.4g Sugars

- 7.6g Protein

INGREDIENTS

- 3 ½ ounces cream cheese, at room temperature

- 1 package smoked salmon, small (.8 oz)

- 2 tbsp. dill, fresh, chopped, plus more for garnishing

- 1/3 cup unsalted butter, at room temperature

- Lettuce leaf, crispy, for serving

- 1 tbsp. lemon juice, fresh

- Pepper to taste

DIRECTIONS

1. Line a large-sized baking sheet with the parchment paper. Combine smoked salmon together with cream cheese, butter, lemon juice, pepper, and dill in a food processor. Pulse on high settings until completely smooth.

2. Spoon approximately 2 tbsp. of the mixture over the lined parchment paper. Garnish with more of dill, if desired.

3. Place the baking sheet in a refrigerator and let chill until set, for 20 to 30 minutes. Serve immediately and enjoy or store them in an airtight container in a refrigerator for up to 1 week.

BAGEL & LOX
FAT BOMBS

Prep Time: 5 minutes
Cooking Time: 35 minutes
Servings: 36 persons

Nutritional Info (Estimated Amount Per Serving)

- 34 Calories

- 21 Calories from Fat

- 2.3g Total Fat

- 1.3g Saturated Fat

- 0g Trans Fat

- 0.1g Polyunsaturated Fat

- 0.6g Monounsaturated Fat

- 7.1mg Cholesterol

- 106mg Sodium

- 19mg Potassium

- 1.9g Total Carbohydrates

- 0.1g Dietary Fiber

- 0.5g Sugars

- 1.3g Protein

INGREDIENTS

- 2 scallions, medium, thinly sliced

- 8 ounces cultured cream cheese, organic

- Everything Bagel Seasoning, homemade

- 4 ounces smoked salmon, wild-caught

DIRECTIONS

1. Beat the cream cheese using a stand or hand mixer, until completely fluffy, for a minute or two.

2. Add in the chopped smoked salmon & then the scallions.

3. Beat again until everything is well incorporated.

4. Now, form bite-sized balls from the mixture and then coat each ball lightly in the homemade seasoning.

5. Let chill in a refrigerator for a couple of hours. Don't forget to thaw before eating.

SALMON AND DILL FAT BOMBS

Prep Time: 5 minutes
Cooking Time: 1 hour & 15 minutes
Servings: 12

Nutritional Info (Estimated Amount Per Serving)

- 163 Calories

- 154 Calories from Fat

- 17g Total Fat

- 10g Saturated Fat

- 0.4g Trans Fat

- 0.7g Polyunsaturated Fat

- 4.5g Monounsaturated Fat

- 48mg Cholesterol

- 262mg Sodium

- 36mg Potassium

- 1.1g Total Carbohydrates

- 0g Dietary Fiber

- 0.7g Sugars

- 1.9g Protein

INGREDIENTS

- ½ package of smoked salmon

- Dill, to taste

- 1 cup cream cheese

- Lemon juice, fresh, to taste

- 2/3 cup butter

- Salt, to taste

DIRECTIONS

1. Add the entire ingredients together in a food processor; blend on high settings.

2. Now, form small-sized balls from the mixture & pop them in a refrigerator. Serve cold and enjoy.

SALMON BENNY BREAKFAST BOMBS

Prep Time: 10 minutes
Cooking Time: 1 hour & 20 minutes
Servings: 2

Nutritional Info (Estimated Amount Per Serving)

- 377 Calories

- 294 Calories from Fat

- 33g Total Fat

- 17g Saturated Fat

- 0.9g Trans Fat

- 2.9g Polyunsaturated Fat

- 10g Monounsaturated Fat

- 396mg Cholesterol

- 1891mg Sodium

- 211mg Potassium

- 1.7g Total Carbohydrates

- 0.3g Dietary Fiber

- 0.5g Sugars

- 19g Protein

INGREDIENTS

For Breakfast Bombs:

- 4 ounces smoked salmon, sliced

- 2 tbsp. chives, fresh, chopped

- ½ tbsp. butter, salted

- 2 eggs, large

- Pepper and salt to taste

For Hollandaise Sauce:

- 2 tsp. freshly squeezed lemon juice

- ¼ tsp. Dijon mustard

- 1 egg yolk, large, separated from the white

- 2 tbsp. salted butter

- Salt to taste

- ½ tbsp. water or more

DIRECTIONS

1. For hollandaise sauce; ensure all the ingredients are at room temperature.

2. Fill a small pot with water and bring it to a boil, over moderate heat settings. Once starts boiling; add 2 eggs; let boil until hard-boiled, for several minutes.

3. In the meantime, finely dice the salmon slices. Make sure that they are separated once cut.

4. Now, over high-heat settings in a large pan; heat 2 tsp. of butter

until completely melted. Once done; add half of the cut up salmon into the pan and cook until crispy; set aside.

5. Once the eggs have boiled for several minutes run them under cold water. Before you start the peeling process; let the eggs to completely cool.

6. When cooled enough, arrange them in a dish and finely mash use a large fork.

7. Now, fill a pot with a few cups of water & bring it to a simmer, over moderate heat settings. Heat 2 tbsp. of butter for 30 to 60 seconds in the microwave, until melted; set aside. Whisk egg yolk together with dijon mustard, lemon juice & a pinch of salt in a heat-safe bowl (preferably large-sized) until air bubbles start to appear. To create a double boiler; place the bowl over the pot with the simmering water. Don't let the bottom to touch the hot water.

8. Continue to whisk the mixture over medium heat settings until it begins to thicken.

9. Slowly pour in the melted butter; continue to stir with a whisk (make sure there are no clumps remaining). Feel free to add some water, if the sauce is too thick. Set aside and let cool at room temperature.

10.   Take the raw salmon, half the chives, prepared hollandaise and mashed egg; mix well until you get a firm mixture like consistency.

11.   Once done, split the mixture evenly into 4 pieces & roll into small-sized balls.

12.   Mix the leftover crispy salmon and chives together & coat the prepared bombs in this mixture.

LOW-CARB PORK CHOPS FAT BOMBS

Prep Time: 10 minutes
Cooking Time: 30 minutes
Servings: 3

Nutritional Info (Estimated Amount Per Serving)

- 506 Calories

- 409 Calories from Fat

- 45g Total Fat

- 5.2g Saturated Fat

- 0.4g Trans Fat

- 7.4g Polyunsaturated Fat

- 30g Monounsaturated Fat

- 59mg Cholesterol

- 51mg Sodium

- 440mg Potassium

- 6.2g Total Carbohydrates

- 1.1g Dietary Fiber

- 2.9g Sugars

- 19g Protein

INGREDIENTS

- 1 tbsp. balsamic vinegar

- 1 tsp. ground nutmeg

- 3 pork chops, medium, boneless

- 1 package brown mushrooms, washed & sliced (8 oz.)

- 1 cup mayonaisse, without added sugar

- 1 tsp. garlic powder

- ½ cup oil

- 1 yellow onion, medium, peeled & sliced

DIRECTIONS

1. Over moderate heat settings in a large skillet, heat the oil and then sauté the onion with mushrooms until wilted, for a couple of minutes.

2. Make some space for the pork chops by pushing the mushrooms and onion aside.

3. Add in the pork chops, and cook until each side turns brown; don't forget to season each chop with nutmeg and garlic powder.

4. Once the pork chops are cooked to your likings, remove them from the pan & let the oil and onions to cool down a bit.

5. Stir in the vinegar and mayo; whisk until combined well and you get a thick, rich sauce.

6. Ladle the prepared sauce on top of the chops. Serve immediately and enjoy.

KETO BACON BURGER BOMBS

Prep Time: 15 minutes
Cooking Time: 20 minutes
Servings: 12

Nutritional Info (Estimated Amount Per Serving)

- 303 Calories

- 241 Calories from Fat

- 27g Total Fat

- 11g Saturated Fat

- 0.3g Trans Fat

- 3.3g Polyunsaturated Fat

- 10g Monounsaturated Fat

- 64mg Cholesterol

- 555mg Sodium

- 154mg Potassium

- 1.5g Total Carbohydrates

- 0g Dietary Fiber

- 0.7g Sugars

- 14g Protein

INGREDIENTS

- 12 rounds sausage patties, raw, (1 ounce)

- 12 bacon slices

- Onion powder, cumin, pepper, salt to taste

- 12 cubes smoked cheddar cheese, (1")

DIRECTIONS

1. Line a cookie sheet with the parchment paper and then preheat your oven to 350 F in advance. Lay your sausage rounds out over the prepared cookie sheet.

2. Dust the sausage with onion powder, cumin, pepper and salt.

3. Place a piece of cheese in the center of the coated sausage rounds.

4. Make a ball with the sausage around the cheese; rolling it in your hands.

5. Wrap the bacon around the sausage balls.

6. Bake in the preheated oven for an hour. Serve immediately and enjoy.

AVOCADO & EGG FAT BOMBS AND DEVILED EGGS

Prep Time: 5 minutes
Cooking Time: 25 minutes
Servings: 5

Nutritional Info (Estimated Amount Per Serving)

- 135 Calories

- 118 Calories from Fat

- 13g Total Fat

- 2.6g Saturated Fat

- 0g Trans Fat

- 5.6g Polyunsaturated Fat

- 4.4g Monounsaturated Fat

- 115mg Cholesterol

- 237mg Sodium

- 103mg Potassium

- 2.4g Total Carbohydrates

- 1.2g Dietary Fiber

- 0.3g Sugars

- 2.5g Protein

INGREDIENTS

- ½ avocado, large, peeled & de-seed

- 1 tbsp. lime or lemon juice

- 3 egg yolks, cooked, large; cut the eggs into half

- Freshly ground black pepper

- ¼ cup mayonnaise

- 2 tbsp. chives or spring onions, chopped

- ½ tsp. Himalayan pink salt or to taste

To Serve:

- Leftover cooked egg white halves

- Freshly cut crispy lettuce leaves, cucumber slices or bell peppers

DIRECTIONS

1. Fill a small pot with water and bring it to a boil, over moderate heat settings. Once starts boiling; add 2 eggs; let boil until hard-boiled, for several minutes.

2. Once the eggs have boiled for several minutes run them under cold water. Before you start the peeling process; let the eggs to completely cool and then peel of their shells.

3. Place the avocado pieces into a food processor & then add in the lemon juice, mayonnaise, egg yolks, pepper and salt. Process on high settings until smooth. Fill up the egg white halves & prepare the deviled eggs. Store for a week in an airtight container. Serve immediately and enjoy.

BREAKFAST BACON FAT BOMBS

Prep Time: 20 minutes
Cooking Time: 35 minutes
Servings: 6

Nutritional Info (Estimated Amount Per Serving)

- 261 Calories
- 238 Calories from Fat
- 26g Total Fat
- 11g Saturated Fat
- 0g Trans Fat
- 3.9g Polyunsaturated Fat
- 10g Monounsaturated Fat
- 75mg Cholesterol
- 220mg Sodium
- 102mg Potassium
- 1g Total Carbohydrates
- 0.4g Dietary Fiber
- 0.4g Sugars
- 4.8g Protein

INGREDIENTS

- 6 bacon slices, cooked

- 1 Serrano pepper, diced & seeded

- ¼ avocado

- 1 egg, large, hardboiled

- 4 tbsp. clarified or unsalted butter

- Juice of ¼ lime, fresh

- 2 tbsp. bacon grease

- 1 tbsp. mayonnaise

- Cracked Pepper & kosher salt, to taste

- 1 tbsp. cilantro, fresh, chopped

DIRECTIONS

1. Combine hardboiled egg together with Serrano pepper, butter, avocado, mayonnaise, and cilantro in a large bowl. Using a potato smasher or fork; mash until you get smooth paste like consistency. Season with pepper and salt, then add in the lime juice; give everything a good stir.

2. Now, cook the bacon until crispy; remove but keeping 2 tbsp. of the bacon grease in the pan. Gently stir bacon grease to the fat bomb mixture. Cover & place in a refrigerator; let chill until you can form solid balls from the mixture, for half an hour. Crumble the bacon in a small bowl into small bits.

3. Make six even-sized balls from the mixture. Add the balls to the bacon bits; rolling the balls around until covered completely. Serve immediately and enjoy.

CHICKEN BOMBS

Prep Time: 15 minutes
Cooking Time: 55 minutes
Servings: 8

Nutritional Info (Estimated Amount Per Serving)

- 305 Calories

- 189 Calories from Fat

- 21g Total Fat

- 7g Saturated Fat

- 0.1g Trans Fat

- 4.9g Polyunsaturated Fat

- 7.3g Monounsaturated Fat

- 46mg Cholesterol

- 518mg Sodium

- 211mg Potassium

- 18g Total Carbohydrates

- 0.7g Dietary Fiber

- 9.3g Sugars

- 11g Protein

INGREDIENTS

- 8 chicken tenders

- 1 package cream cheese, softened (8 ounce)

- 6 tbsp. pepper jelly

- ¼ cup green onion, finely chopped or to taste

- 8 bacon slices

- 1 finely chopped jalapeno pepper

- Ground black pepper and salt to taste

DIRECTIONS

1. Set a wire rack over the baking sheet and preheat your oven to 400 F in advance.

2. Combine green onion together with cream cheese, jalapeno pepper, pepper, and salt in a large bowl.

3. Using the flat side of a meat tenderizer; pound the chicken tenders into a rectangular shape. Place approximately 3 tbsp. of the cream cheese mixture in center of each tender and then fold into a pouch.

4. Now, wrap a bacon slice around each pouch; securing everything with a toothpick and then top with a small quantity of pepper jelly. Place them on the prepared wire rack.

5. Bake for 30 to 35 minutes, until chicken juices run clear and bacon is crisp.

www.ingramcontent.com/pod-product-compliance
Lightning Source LLC
Chambersburg PA
CBHW070113260726

48658CB00001B/98